The New Evolution Diet

The New Evolution Diet

What Our Paleolithic Ancestors Can Teach Us about Weight Loss, Fitness, and Aging

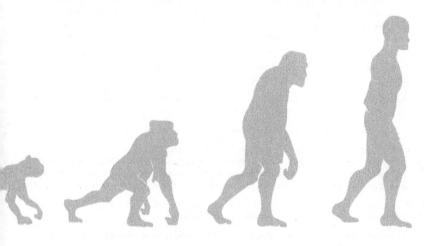

Arthur De Vany, Ph.D.

with an Afterword by Nassim Nicholas Taleb, author of *Fooled by Randomness*

This book is dedicated to my wonder woman,
my wife, Carmela De Vany,
whose energy, love, and humor inspire and nourish me.

Contents

Acknowledgments

A few key people and events do change your life. I owe much to my many and enthusiastic blog readers. They have taught me much and their success stories inspire me every day. I would not have written this book without their inspiration. Bryan Appleyard's article about me and "the diet that really works" in the *Times* of London was a turning point in the progression of this work. His 28-pound weight loss on the New Evolution Diet is his reward. Had Nassim Nicholas Taleb not introduced Bryan to me, this book might not exist. Thanks, Nassim, for creating this "black swan" event, and thanks, Bryan, for so accurately and passionately capturing the essentials of my evolutionary approach. I deeply appreciate the enthusiasm and commitment of my U.S. publisher, Rodale, for this revolutionary concept of diet and lifestyle. My editor there, Julie Will, offered comments and useful advice at every turn and her support and enthusiasm for this book were infectious. I thank my agent, Richard Pine, for being such a reliable and supportive guide through the publication maze. My super editor, Bill Tonelli, crafted my academic writing into the highly accessible and graceful prose you see here on every page. Thanks, Bill, and my readers thank you.

Introduction

Behind the New Evolution Diet

Charles Darwin was overweight and chronically ill. So what can we learn from him about health and fitness?

His theory of evolution clears away a lot of the nonsense we hear these days about how to control our weight and get in shape. It also provides us with a powerful model for understanding why we gain weight and lose strength and vitality as we age. Understanding human evolution provides us with a path we can take to become healthier and happier.

So, what *does* fitness (or the lack of it) have to do with evolution?

This book is the culmination of my decades-long study of weight, diet, and health, which has come to be known as Evolutionary Fitness (and has evolved into the New Evolution Diet). In it, I attempt to offer guidance in these matters, based in part on what life was like roughly 40,000 years ago.

This is not out of any nostalgia I have for the Stone Age but is rather an acknowledgment that, as far as our bodies are concerned, nothing much has changed since then.

So, who were we 40,000 years ago? Our ancestors of that era were tall, muscular, and lean. Food was often scarce. Exercise (meaning the physical activity required to survive) was made up of heavy labor plus intense but brief "fight-or-flight" emergencies. Our ancestors retained their health throughout their lives, though their life spans were considerably shorter than ours because of greater incidences of infection, infant mortality, predators, and accidents.

Homo erectus, our ancestor from almost 2 million years ago, could go out today and buy a suit (42 long) at Ralph Lauren and walk the streets of New York with little notice. He would be tall and lean, built like an NBA guard. A more modern Cro-Magnon, who roamed the earth 40,000 years ago, might buy an Armani (44 long)—he would have a better sense of style than *Homo erectus,* as evidenced in the art objects and cave paintings he left behind. A Cro-Magnon might look more like a rugby player; he would be taller than most males now and would be lean, muscular, and very powerful—a devastating athlete. He would also have a bigger brain than we have. All this can be inferred from Cro-Magnon skeletons, from the capabilities of contemporary hunter-gatherers, and through comparisons between other animals living in the laboratory and in the wild.

Similarly, a female Cro-Magnon would be slender and a bit taller than a modern female, with the classic hourglass shape and posture of a graceful woman. Based on the depictions of shapely females found in Cro-Magnon art, she might look like a supermodel, but not a skinny, starved waif—more Cindy Crawford than Kate Moss.

Modern humans carry a copy of the same genes as our Cro-Magnon ancestors from 28,000 years ago. At least 70 percent of European humans alive today can trace their genes to the small band of Cro-Magnon humans who managed to survive the last Ice Age. The origins of the seven tribes of humans living in Europe can be traced to seven males who lived between 100,000 BC and 40,000 BC. [1]

Why, then, does this same genetic material, which once expressed health and muscular leanness in our ancestors, now express obesity and chronic illness? The answer, of course, is the environment in which our genes express themselves—meaning our modern, affluent society.

In short, we are genetically engineered to thrive in a different world. I believe that if you took prehistoric hunter-gatherers and placed them in our environment, they would behave just as we do and would eventually suffer the same problems. We know this is true because we are hunter-gatherers and we do suffer. We also know that when contemporary hunter-gatherers enter industrialized society, they end up with our bad habits and chronic ailments. [2]

This brings us to a key concept to keep in mind as you read on: We humans evolved when food was scarce and life was full of arduous physical activity. Hence, our bodies instruct us to eat everything we can lay our hands on and to exert ourselves as little as possible.

That's right. We are, in essence, hardwired to be lazy overeaters.

This was a perfect strategy for success thousands of years ago. No human could survive in 40,000 BC unless he or she ate anytime food was available. Our ancestors knew that famine was always close at hand—feast now or suffer tomorrow. They were also careful to expend as little energy as possible, because burning more calories than absolutely necessary was a threat to survival. There were unpredictable intervals of low food intake, even occasional starvation, interwoven with times of abundance.

In the modern world, a hunter-gatherer would follow those same principles: He'd eat a lot and move a little. And he would suffer the same ills we do, living in a modern environment where food is abundant and physical activity is more or less voluntary. Most diet and exercise plans ask us to move more and eat less—a direct contradiction of our genetically engineered impulses. No wonder most diets don't work.

Our forager ancestors also sought out high-energy (meaning high-calorie, high-fat) foods that could be obtained at the lowest energy cost. They would eat or not depending on what they could find or kill, meaning mealtime was a fairly unpredictable thing. They would move when hungry (or when being pursued) and relax once fed—like wild animals do today. Their physical activity would be sporadic, meaning short bursts of intense activity (hunting, hauling, climbing, running) separated by long stretches of languid rest and play. This is the environment for which our behaviors and our metabolism are designed. For all our genes can tell, this is still the way of the world. Only we know different.

Why *do* we get fat and sick? This is an odd question from an evolutionary perspective, because ancestral humans were not overweight. Nor did they suffer the ailments that are so prevalent in our civilized world. We began getting heavier and developing new diseases once we ceased to live as hunter-gatherers and instead became farmers (or more specifically, once we started eating the food we grow rather than gathering food).

Now we suffer from a host of chronic "Western" diseases that were virtually unknown among our early ancestors and are largely absent even among today's hunter-gatherers living in traditional ways. The list is long and depressingly familiar: obesity, adult-onset (type 2) diabetes, high blood pressure, heart disease, Alzheimer's, and on and on.

The origin of these modern ailments can be linked, to some degree, to problems with human metabolism and inflammation. Something in modern life is disturbing the internal systems that evolution handed down to us.

In general, our bodies do not thrive on modern life, where inactivity is imposed by desk jobs and where alcohol, drugs (prescription and otherwise), and even food are abused. Nor do our minds seem to enjoy contemporary living. Humans today likely experience more chronic stress than did our ancestors, whose stresses would have been acute and episodic. The fight-or-flight instincts our ancestors relied on to escape danger are triggered in us today by innumerable and certainly less grave circumstances that have no resolution. The resulting chronic stress is a potent source of misery and disease. Even our wealth and possessions cannot ease this never-ending stress—and in fact, often seem to exacerbate it.

You can see the evolutionary history of our species in the development of the human fetus. The child in gestation looks like a minnow at first, then like a tadpole, then like a frog or maybe a large shrimp. Little buds poke out where limbs develop; the ribs of the fishlike skeleton fuse to form a pelvis; the head enlarges and eye buds pop out, and the fetus starts to resemble a pale, curled-up dolphin. Only gradually does the fetus develop into something that looks human.

A human baby born today would just as easily thrive 40,000 years ago, and a baby born in 40,000 BC would look just like a baby born today. They would have the same genes and develop into normal children and adults in either era. Each child born today carries genes that prepare him or her for the life of a hunter-gatherer, the occupation of every human who has ever lived except for those of us who were born after the recent invention of agriculture 10,000 years ago.

The remarkable thing is that we do so well in the modern world. That little baby born today has no more genetic instructions on how to live and survive now than the one born 40,000 years ago had. Today's baby is no stronger, smarter, or better suited for life than one who was born in the distant past. Even though Paleolithic children grew up to make stone chips and spears and to hunt mammoth, they used the same neural pathways and learning skills that allow modern children to grow up to make computer chips and business deals. They have the same brain and the same body and can therefore have the same thoughts, and with enough training, can do the same things. They are different only because they live in different worlds, and there is the rub.

That baby whose genes, brain, and body expect him or her to be a forager grows up to be a sales manager or a tax accountant. Instead of

roaming the African savanna scrounging for food, she shops in a supermarket. Rather than pursuing antelope, he tracks financial flows on a
spreadsheet. And certainly, neither of their ancestors ever craved a
french fry or drank a soda.

Many of the foods we eat today are completely novel substances
from an evolutionary perspective. The human preference for sweet
tastes is an evolutionary adaptation—a capability or trait that confers a
particular advantage in a specific environment—that developed in an
environment where such treats were rare and signaled dense, useful
energy. For instance, hunter-gatherers (then and now) prize honey and
risk the wrath of wild bees to capture this sweet. Fruits were only seasonally available to our ancestors, so when they found them, they
tended to eat all they could gather. This once-helpful preference for
sugar is the downfall of many a dieter today. It's what makes it hard to
resist sweets, especially when they are all around us.

But even if some of our evolutionary adaptations no longer work to
our advantage, our quality of life today is better than ever. We are safer
and more comfortable, and we are all but free of the many pathogens
and parasites that threatened our ancestors. Far fewer infants die now
than did in the Paleolithic or Old Stone Age. Life expectancy is higher
not only at birth but also at all ages now (although not by as much as
you might expect in the later years).[3]

Our ancestors had a higher probability of death at every age than we
do, but they lived a smaller portion of their lives in disability. Modern
humans live longer but age more rapidly than our prehistoric ancestors,
and we live more of our lives in chronic illness. (Though this, arguably,
is better than not living at all.) Our forebears were fit well into their
advanced years. They aged well. A good deal of what we call normal
aging is a modern condition that is more akin to disease than any natural state of growing older.

There is a reason for this. In scientific jargon, we are active *genotypes*
trying to live as sedentary *phenotypes*. In plain English: We are not living as we were built to live. Our genes were forged in an environment

where activity was mandatory—creating a strong selective pressure for genes that encoded a smart, physically adept individual capable of very high activity levels. Historically, humans have ranked among the most active animal species, and we carry energetically expensive brains to boot. The sedentary phenotype, *Homo sedentarius,* is the typical modern human who gets no exercise, becomes overweight or obese, is unfit and chronically ill, and ages rapidly. He ignores his biological need for activity. Inactivity and obesity alter the expression of our genes, making us more susceptible to an array of modern debilitating ailments.

So regular exercise is not just something you do to improve your health and drop a little weight. It is not an "intervention," as some health professionals call it. It is absolutely essential to a healthy life—as necessary as food, water, and air. You exercise because the length and quality of your life depend on it.

What happens to astronauts in space is pretty convincing evidence of the necessity of physical activity. The space traveler's body wastes away when it is subjected to a zero-gravity environment. In fact, astronauts must exercise in space or they are likely to become ill by the end of a long mission. And even though they do work out, many astronauts have returned to Earth having lost a good deal of their muscle, organ, heart, and skeletal tissue (probably brain tissue, too).[4]

A couch astronaut does no less damage; it just takes longer for him to waste away. The lean body mass of the couch astronaut disappears even as his circumference, total body mass, and body fat percentage grow. This altered body composition will age him rapidly because he is also losing his metabolic fitness.

The good news in all this is that our genes are not the sum total of our destiny; we can alter our gene expression for better or worse.

One thing we can do in that regard is to eat properly. A forager moving over the savanna in the quest for food will encounter patches of edible plants in great variety and in seasonal abundance. Even in the marginal environments that contemporary hunter-gatherers occupy, as many as 300 edible plants may grow seasonally. We are adapted to consume a large and changing variety of foods. In fact, people who eat a variety of foods experience superior health and longevity compared with those who eat a monotonous diet composed of the same few staples.[5]

As with food, variety in activity is beneficial to health. I believe we should model our physical activity after the movements of children at play or predators at work. This leads to a rather radical but peaceful departure from a good deal of common advice regarding exercise.

I take life easier than almost anyone I know, but when I do exercise, I move as though my life depends on it—which it does. I never work out more than an hour and a half per week, and I sometimes go days without exercising at all. I spend more time doing nothing than most people I know—really nothing, not reading or watching television, just taking easy walks with my wife, or roaming the hills near our home, or lying on the grass with my dogs and watching the sky. I even organize my work life that way, mixing intensely productive periods with stretches of pure laziness.

A forager may spend many fruitless hours in search of high-energy animal foods, subsisting on plants until the next kill. I think human metabolism is adapted to this pattern of intermittent variety in food sources and periodic fasting mixed with varying activity levels. The chronic routine of three balanced meals and two snacks a day combined with the chronic routine of repetitive exercise just does not square with how our metabolism is built to function. There must be a periodic emptying of energy reserves through activity and intermittent hunger. Unless we do this, I don't think it is possible to overcome the instinct to eat more than we burn that allowed our hunter-gatherer ancestors to survive and pass their genes on to us.

A large body of genetic research supports this view, as I will discuss in various places throughout the book. The same research supports the view that it is the grain-based carbohydrate in our diets that hinders our metabolism from functioning as evolution intended.

Darwin wrote, "Reproduction is how life commutes its death sentence." What he meant was that our DNA has to decide whether our genes will repair themselves or depend on our sexual reproduction to carry our genes forward. During times of plenty, our DNA allows us to reproduce. When resources are scarce, it focuses on self-repair, which extends our good health and longevity. DNA takes its signal from carbohydrate—if it exists in abundance, our DNA assumes that food is plentiful, and so it can rely on our reproduction impulses. That mechanism is a powerful reason for restricting our carb intake—doing so may trigger our self-repair processes. It may also help us to control our weight.

The strategies of the New Evolution Diet are simple and powerful. Here are the guiding principles:

- **Enjoy the pleasure of food and do not count or restrict calories.** Eat a diet low in glucose and starch that is similar (but not identical) to the one humans lived with for thousands of years as human metabolism evolved. Glucose restriction offers antiaging benefits, too.

- **Do not starve yourself, but *do* go hungry episodically, for brief periods.** This means you should practice partial fasting once a week or so. An easy way to fast is to skip a meal when you have something else to do.

- **Exercise less, not more, but with greater playfulness and intensity.** Exercise for the pleasure of the sensation, not to burn calories. Exercise to create a beautiful, strong body with a high resting metabolism and a large physiologic capacity that will help you move through life easily and handle stress and challenges easily.

By giving up on the traditional yet unsuccessful "eat less, exercise more" approach to health, you will suffer far less stress. By varying your eating patterns, the foods you eat, and your activities, you will transform your chronic, debilitating stress into episodes of brief, energizing, acute stress that are actually beneficial.

By exercising more like a wild animal than like a robot, you will build a physical capacity that brings a kind of fearlessness and a sense of confidence that you are up to any situation you may face. Brief, more-intense exercise supplies energy to the brain to offset hunger in a way that long and slow exercise cannot.

Muscle is medicine; it releases many substances that promote health. Body fat is poison; it sends forth chemicals that disrupt metabolism and promote chronic disease and aging. Building muscle alters our metabolism; as we increase muscle mass, energy and nutrients are directed to our brain and muscle—not to our fat stores. When you become more slender and muscular, your body composition (ratio of muscle to fat) makes it easy to maintain weight in a stable range.

There is no need for willpower on this diet because you do not need to restrict calories. The number on the scale is meaningless. The New Evolution Diet is not about losing weight—it's about helping you achieve a healthy balance of muscle and fat.

Sounds easy? That's because it *is*. Please allow me to show you.

CHAPTER 1

My Journey

It seems as though I have been researching this book all my life.

I began lifting weights and taking an interest in diet at the age of 14. As I have heard many others say, it all began in a garage with a 90-pound weight set. My gains came quickly, so at 16 I joined a gym operated by John Farbotnik, a former Mr. America. John's gym was a hangout for Olympic athletes from the Pasadena Athletic Club, and I wanted to be around them. I weighed 196 pounds at age 16 (almost 60 years later I weigh about the same) and began lifting in the demanding Olympic style because it was more athletic than what I had been doing.

I had hopes of playing professional baseball and felt that the speed and power I developed through weight training were what I needed to gain a competitive edge. It was a good move because few ballplayers then lifted, and it made me strong and quick. I signed a contract with the Hollywood Stars, a minor league team that was part of the Pittsburgh Pirates organization, right out of high school. But my eyesight and ambitions got the better of my baseball career. I went on to UCLA, where I got my Ph.D. in economics. After a few years working in think tanks, I became an academic so I could follow my own research interests.

I was primarily interested in studying what was *not* known in my field, which took me into the realm of complex systems, wild variations, and extreme events—the so-called black swans that author Nassim Nicholas Taleb writes about. This led me back to Hollywood, not to play baseball but to study the movie business and how it adapted to uncertainty. I didn't know it at the time, but this was excellent preparation for the study of metabolism. I wrote a book about the economics of Hollywood and settled into the University of California, Irvine Department of Economics and Institute for Mathematical Behavioral Sciences for the last 20 years of my academic career.

My education in metabolism began the year I was a visiting scholar at the University of Chicago, during the blizzard of '79. My youngest son, Brandon, had developed type 1 diabetes, probably from a viral infection that triggered a strong immune response. The doctors believed that my son's pancreas suffered collateral damage from the firepower his immune system aimed at the virus. When this happens, insulin secretion in the important beta cells of the pancreas stops or is severely depressed.

Only type 1 diabetics suffer this autoimmunity, for reasons that are still unclear. There is a genetic link—my wife, Bonnie, later developed diabetes, too—but something has to trigger the expression of the genes that cause this excessive response from the immune system. My guess is that both my wife and son had very active and aggressive immune systems, since they almost never got sick. In Brandon's and Bonnie's cases, their immune systems permanently altered their metabolisms.

Because I was an academic at heart, I responded to my son's medical crisis by going to the university bookstore. I bought books on diabetes and metabolism and a large textbook on endocrinology that I owned until a few months ago, when I donated it to the local library. I learned as much as I could about insulin and diabetes. Eventually, I knew enough to discuss these topics intelligently with Brandon's doctors, and even to engage them in friendly debate about various treatments and appropriate insulin injection doses.

Food was our most contentious topic. My son's doctors wanted him to eat cereal or pancakes with syrup and orange juice for breakfast, sandwiches or pasta for lunch with Jell-O for dessert, and beans or potatoes and low-fat meats for dinner. Carbs were friendly, the doctors maintained, and fat was the enemy. Doughnuts were fine and starches were healthy. The American Diabetes Association still recommends a relatively high-carb, low-saturated-fat diet some thirty years later.

But it was evident to me that my son was not eating the right foods. He was getting too much carbohydrate and injecting too much insulin to manage the load it imposed on his damaged metabolism. Each dose of carbohydrate had to be followed by an injection of insulin or his blood glucose would rise too high. But if we injected too much insulin, his glucose level would drop dangerously, and he would become jittery and angry. If this condition worsens, it can lead to unconsciousness and death. Brandon would sometimes even refuse to take a glucose tablet, a problem many diabetics experience as their blood glucose drops and they become emotional and stubborn. Their brains, in glucose crisis, descend into primitive behavior and lose control of rational decision making.

As you may know, insulin's job is to extract glucose (a form of sugar) from the bloodstream to store it for later use. But things go wrong when this hormone performs its task too well. It will actually withhold glucose from the bloodstream even when the brain is being denied this essential fuel and nears unconsciousness. The other hormones that can also mobilize energy are powerless to help. The brain in those instances *could* extract the glucose it needs from elsewhere in the body, mainly from the liver and muscle—except that the insulin overrides the hormones (glucagon and cortisol) responsible for that task. Insulin is essential but also potentially dangerous; it is the instrument of choice in movies (and sometimes, in reality) when a doctor wants to murder his wife or a rogue nurse wants to kill patients.

I knew as an economist that it made no sense to try to manage blood glucose, which is a flow, with a storage hormone like insulin. Eating carbohydrates and then hoping to inject just the right amount of insulin to utilize the glucose was a crude, imprecise approach to disease management. It was bound to make my son gain excess weight, because safety required that he consume more sugar than he needed, lest his brain get too little glucose and go into shock.

Eventually, we got off the carbs-insulin seesaw. But not just yet.

My education in metabolism was furthered when my wife, Bonnie, also developed type 1 diabetes, 12 years after Brandon. We weren't sure why this happened, and neither were her doctors—type 2 diabetes is the form of the disease typically referred to as "adult-onset." My hunch was that she had been taking too much thyroid medicine, which stressed her metabolism to the breaking point. We had better tools for diabetics by then; meters had become simple and inexpensive, so we could measure her blood glucose more accurately than we could Brandon's when he was diagnosed.

Bonnie ate as her doctors suggested because she loved pasta, potatoes, pancakes, and bread. But injecting insulin to manage her starchy diet made her gain weight, too, and soon she was doing her best to balance between too little insulin and too much. We experienced many terrifying nights with Bonnie deep in insulin shock as I tried to get some glucose into her.

I began to examine Bonnie's testing numbers and correlate her blood glucose with her meals. I used my training in statistics to look for patterns in her readings; I wanted to see if I could find the triggers for her worst episodes of insulin shock and high glucose. I tried to determine which foods increased her blood glucose and how much insulin was necessary to bring it back down to a healthy level.

It soon became apparent that striving to keep blood glucose in a narrow range using insulin injections was counterproductive, even dangerous; this is a conclusion that current research also supports. It is now well recognized that tight glucose control improves a few markers of damage from hyperglycemia, but is associated with higher mortality. Both my wife and my son experienced too many episodes of low blood glucose that put them in or close to insulin shock. These ordeals were exhausting for them. They became depressed and gained weight. Brandon, who had been lean, became a chubby boy. Bonnie, who had been a slim *Vogue* cover girl, put on weight and then dropped it again in cycles. She still was beautiful, but the stress was taking its toll.

It became clear that each drastic rise and fall in their blood glucose level increased the likelihood of similar events happening down the line. This suggested that the brain has a metabolic memory that records events and responds in similar ways when they occur again. The brain was learning to make the adjustments necessary to bring blood glucose into a stable range. But soon it was overreacting, like a driver oversteering as he tries to control a swerving car. The cycle of swinging back and forth is itself dangerous. Some type 1 diabetics become what doctors call "brittle," meaning that they swing too easily from high to low blood glucose levels.

We needed to teach the brain a better strategy. I believed we had to let the brain learn to mobilize glucose from sources *inside* the body instead of relying on external supplies, meaning carbs. We had to use less insulin, and to do that we had to eat fewer foods that raised blood glucose.

The New Evolution Diet developed directly out of our experiments with food and Bonnie's response to them. She tested her blood glucose after each meal, and then we examined the data to see what had triggered an elevation in that level and how much insulin was needed to bring it back to a healthy range.

Pasta and potatoes sent her blood glucose through the roof, requiring a large injection of insulin to bring it back down. So pasta and potatoes were the first entries on our list of offending dishes. We identified all such foods and simply cut them out. We did not just reduce her intake of these foods—we banished them. I did not want her reactivating old metabolic memories by eating small amounts of offending dishes. The list of forbidden foods grew over time, and our mealtimes became an experiment: We'd test the reaction of her blood glucose to a specific food and note the amount of insulin that was needed to bring it back to a healthy range. We did not know it at the time, but 25 years ago we were creating our own glycemic index, which is used to determine acceptable carbohydrates for the Zone diet, the South Beach Diet, and many other popular eating regimens.

Right behind pasta and potatoes, bread and beans made the list of banned foods, because they, too, prompted a large rise in blood glucose. Breakfast cereal and cinnamon buns, Bonnie's favorite, went on the list next.

The program was a success. Soon, a minimal amount of insulin was needed to keep my wife and son stable. One doctor refused to believe Bonnie was a diabetic because she was injecting so little insulin.

Today it is generally accepted that there's a strong link between diabetes and obesity. Overweight people (even nondiabetics) are often insulin-resistant, meaning their bodies don't respond properly to the existing insulin levels, and so they require more of the hormone. An important cause of insulin resistance among type 2 diabetics is the inflammation that is caused by elevated blood glucose and excess body fat. So you see, fat isn't just this stuff inside your body that expands your waistline. It is metabolically active tissue with organlike capabilities. Fat secretes hormones that make other tissues resist the action of insulin. An overweight person requires more insulin than a slender person to manage glucose.

The fresh vegetables and fruit we were consuming drastically reduced my wife's inflammation as she lost weight and excess body fat. In response, her insulin sensitivity increased. Best of all, we ate wonderfully on our new diet. We didn't feel the least bit deprived. After a while, it didn't require any self-control, which is a good thing for several reasons. Most people don't realize that acts of self-control are such hard mental work that they actually deplete the glucose levels in the brain. Therefore, you will lack willpower when glucose is low or cannot be mobilized effectively. It's a big reason why dieting doesn't work.

As Bonnie's stress level was reduced, her brain's metabolic memories of past trauma began to fade. Her neural networks had reformed as the old ones faded for lack of use. In fact, at this point all of our bodies had adjusted—so much so that eating any of the offending substances left us feeling sick and bloated.

From then on, I cooked dinner quite a lot, which was a new experience for me. I had previously been on the relatively high-carbohydrate diet that was popular in athletic circles. I recall seeing pictures of Olympic athletes "carbing out" before events by eating big platefuls of pasta. I had never eaten that way on a daily basis, but before a big athletic event I would often load up on starches. Now I had to learn to eat differently.

I would stop at the store on the way home from work and browse the produce section, looking for something fresh and colorful. Then I would go to the seafood or meat aisle for some healthy protein before heading home to make dinner with whatever I had found. My shopping trips were confined to the periphery of the supermarket, meaning I seldom ventured into the center aisles, where the processed and packaged foods are located. I usually would cook more than we could eat at one meal, so we could have breakfast, lunch, or another dinner from the leftovers. It was faster than fast food. Much better and cheaper, too.

So this was a breakthrough for us, but it was still just our little family project. Then one day in my office, I was talking with an anthropology graduate student who had come in to discuss a project she was working on, which explored reciprocity between members of a tribe.

We talked about meat sharing, and I brought up our new diet. I told her that my family and I had begun eating only fresh vegetables, fruits, nuts, seafood, and meat. She told me that the tribal members she studied ate the same way. It should have been obvious to me, but I hadn't thought about it: I had come up with a typical hunter-gatherer meal plan.

Intrigued, I made the rounds among my anthropologist colleagues at the institute to discuss this and to ask what I should read on the subject. I found it ironic that these people who knew so much about hunter-gatherers all ate a high-carb diet. Many of the scholars were overweight. I thought, if they know so much about the human mind and its evolution, why are they so heavy? I think they had separated their knowledge of science from their personal habits, as many people seem to do, but gave little thought to what they ate.

I began to study the human genome, the library of our genes. The modern human genome is about 50,000 to 100,000 years old. Little has changed during that time except for some variation in the genes that adapt to disease, as well as some adaptive changes that have been made as a result of our nutrition—such as the ability to metabolize the sugar lactose contained in milk.

I began to look into the relationship between the original human diet that was consumed by hunter-gatherers and our genetic makeup. I focused on 40,000 BC, when fully modern humans emerged. The diet they consumed was strikingly similar to what my family and I had developed in our attempt to control diabetes.

The current debate over fat versus carbohydrate is anchored totally in the modern idea of eating. This is really an argument over fads, because virtually every modern diet is just a small variation on bad nutritional thinking. Excellent research has been done on this topic by many scholars, notably Loren Cordain, whose book, *The Paleo Diet: Lose Weight and Get Healthy by Eating the Food You Were Designed to Eat,* provides helpful guidance on the hunter-gatherer lifestyle.[1]

I came to think of our family diet, derived through careful experimentation with the foods that exist today, as a modern form of the "original" diet. We were not trying to mimic the Paleolithic diet, or to "eat paleo," as the expression goes. It's not necessary to do anything so drastic. I think our genes can handle contemporary life just fine if we

help them with diet and activity. In fact, I believe that the current epi-
demics of insulin resistance and metabolic disease are really an attempt
by our genes to keep us alive and healthy on a diet that misdirects our
metabolism.

Oddly, it was my understanding of decentralized economic systems
and their use of price to guide the allocation of resources that led me to
address the big question of human metabolism: How does your body
know where and when to send energy and nutrients? Inside, you are
not a single organism—you are a vast colony of trillions of cells bound
in a complex dance of cooperation and competition that somehow sus-
tains life. There is no centralized control. Each cell has its genetic program whose expression is influenced by its neighbors and its
development sequence in such a way that one cell can be liver tissue
and another can be cardiac muscle.

To borrow a term from economics, our cells are specialized. They
perform their individual functions in response to the neural, hormonal,
and other signals they receive from their surroundings. Good health is
possible only if our cells follow these signals correctly. Disease, cell
damage, and many other insults result from miscommunication and
destroy the internal order that is required to keep us alive and healthy.

As we've discussed, those genes evolved at a time when humans
lived in a world vastly different from today's. We are genetically built
to thrive on a 40,000-year-old diet. The further we stray from that, the
more we endanger our health.

But eating was only half the puzzle. I took my economics analogy
further, applying the dynamical statistical models I developed in my
research to the movement of wild animals, children at play, and sports
events. I would eventually use this model to understand the complex
energy dynamics of Paleolithic hunter-gatherers as they foraged for
food. There were periods of feast and famine and mixtures of physical
activity that varied enormously in intensity and duration.

Hunger motivates movement. This is a genetically engineered survival tactic. If you are starved, you have a powerful reason to get up

and do something about it. That's a good moment to exercise, if you're interested in getting maximum results. A researcher once told me he could not get his lab rats to do their mandatory exercise unless they were hungry. One well-fed rat would just sit on the treadmill and let the wheel rub the fur of its behind—we all know people like that.

What was most revealing about trying to model the Paleolithic energy environment was how our ancestors moved. A hunter had to walk long distances, sprint, and then, in the kill, had to execute abrupt, violent motions. If the hunt was successful, he'd have to lift and haul a heavy load back home. A gatherer, too, walked far, depending on what she sought, and then had to return home bearing a burden. Most of life was random and unpredictable. There was no such thing as a "typical" activity. A hunter expended energy in great bursts of activity and treks of varying length, but then, a lot of the time, did absolutely nothing.

From that insight, it was a short leap to begin exercising in a new way. I began doing intermittent, high-intensity workouts to emulate what I thought prehistoric man would have had to do in the course of his normal existence. There is now abundant research that shows that short bursts of high-intensity exercise yield better results than the monotonous routine of moderately taxing, hyper-regimented exercise. I began to exercise *less* than ever before, but harder. I didn't follow a standard workout routine—I never did the same exercises in the same order twice. I still lifted, pushed, pulled, and reached, but as the spirit moved me, not according to a "plan." I also varied the time of day I exercised and the amount of time between workouts. I might spend a few minutes in the gym one day, an hour the next time, and then stay away altogether for a day or two, to give myself time to recover. Sometimes I'd just find a field nearby and try to simulate some brief but intense "fight-or-flight" moments, as if I were chasing something (or something was chasing me).

It worked splendidly. Already muscular and lean, I hit new levels of both. A famous sculptress asked me to pose for her (I was in my late sixties at the time), and I noticed that other people at the gym started to watch me work out. Some approached me and asked what I ate and did to achieve such impressive results. They never believed me when I shared my philosophy, because it was contrary to everything they "knew" about fitness.

My diet and exercise had altered my metabolism to express my inner hunter-gatherer. I had become a 21st-century caveman.

And that was my private journey, which soon became a public one through a suitably 21st-century method: my blog.

That began in a somewhat roundabout way. I already had a university Web site, devoted to my courses and studies in economics. Then, in the early '90s, I decided to put into writing all that I had learned about health, in an essay titled "Evolutionary Fitness." As an afterthought, I posted it on the site and then put up more writings on health, diet, and fitness. I was surprised by all the e-mail responses I received from readers who were as fascinated with the subject as I was.

In 2003, after I retired from the university, I established a blog of my own. I posted some articles that had been written about my work on movie economics (the best was in *The New Yorker*, a piece by John Cassidy titled "Chaos in Hollywood: Can Science Explain Why a Movie Is a Hit or a Flop?"). Like Nassim Nicholas Taleb, I was by then studying the consequences of extreme events on economics and elsewhere, and I put that research on the blog, too.

Eventually, my studies led me to realize that extreme events even affect human metabolism. There is now a huge amount of research establishing this point of view, and you will find the essence of that somewhat complicated approach to health discussed later in the book. It is overly intellectualized, no doubt, but it does lead to some very simple insights, the main one being that life itself is driven far more by extreme events than by the steady drip of the average.

In matters of health, we tend to use the words *average* and *normal* almost interchangeably. But mathematicians and other "numbers people" know that the average can sometimes be meaningless; a common joke on the subject is that if half the world's population is male, then humans have an average of one testicle each. Sometimes, "average" is just the midpoint between extreme highs and lows. When discussing health, those extremes can be equally unhealthy, and so being average may be unhealthy, too.

The average level of insulin, for example, has drifted upward over time as more and more people are diagnosed with hyperinsulinemia, so that to be "normal" now in this regard is not a good thing. It may just mean you are as unhealthy as your neighbor. The average testosterone level of males has declined over the past two decades. That's another realm where I would rather not be average.

The concern for balancing the average intake of food and output of energy is also misplaced, in my opinion. No living creature ever lived in perfect energy balance, where calorie input and output were always exactly equal. The diet experts would have you strive for such a state. But it's a totally unnatural way to live, impossible to maintain, anxiety-causing, and not much fun. Even if you could live that way, it wouldn't make you healthy.

I posted my research on these topics and much to my surprise, traffic on my blog grew rather rapidly. I had never advertised or sought out search engines or done any of the things people do now in order to draw Web site visitors. The blog seemed to be a self-organizing process. New traffic tended to generate still more new traffic, and at times the growth was explosive. By 2006 the traffic had become so great that I had to shift to high-speed servers to keep up with the demand.

I think it was the array of topics that I discussed and my rather unusual perspective that attracted readers. Remarkably, it drew a substantial number of scientists and researchers in various fields related to economics, finance, health, and fitness. I also noticed that a number of distinguished research institutions' Web sites included links to my blog.

Month after month there were visitors from 115 different countries. I made friends all over the world just sitting at my computer, writing down my thoughts.

Early on, my health-related postings began to attract attention. In 1999 a PBS program called *Closer to Truth* called to see if I would appear on an episode titled "Can You Really Extend Your Life?" I joined a distinguished group—the host, Dr. Robert Lawrence Kuhn; Dr. Sherwin Nuland, the Yale professor and bestselling author; Dr. French Anderson, one of the early pioneers of gene therapy; and Dr. Roy Walford, a pioneering life-extension researcher and author of *The 120 Year Diet*.

I think I surprised the other guests, who had probably assumed I would be a kook. But none of the other guests raised the issue I did: At the same time that they were talking about life extension, we were seeing a progressive *loss* of health and longevity in the United States. Little or none of the perspective these wise men offered seemed to have reached the rest of the country. If anything, healthy life expectancy was declining with the rise of metabolic syndrome, diabetes, and obesity, thanks to a terrible diet, a lack of exercise, and metabolic disease. Our high-minded academic discussion about the possibilities of life extension and improving health quality had little to do with reality.

The host, Dr. Kuhn, said that merely doing the show was stressful. Apparently it was, because he ate nervously throughout the taping. The spread laid out for the guests included sweet rolls, muffins, and other simple carbs, and even candy bars. When I told this brilliant man that he was eating so much junk because his insulin was too high and that mixing insulin with stress hormones caused stress eating, he was taken aback. I disagreed with the diet and exercise advice he promulgated— eat your grains and do your cardio—and told him so. Why emphasize grains, I asked, when they cause insulin resistance, provoke the immune system, damage the gut, and contain too many simple carbohydrates? He had no answer. Whether his attitude or diet changed, I cannot say, since I lost contact with him. Sadly, my fellow guest Dr. Walford, the life-extension guru, did not live to be 120; he died just 3 years later.

My ideas have found a particularly hospitable home in Great Britain, thanks in part to a newspaper story that was done about me in the *Times* of London in 2008. In it, the writer Bryan Appleyard described me in a way that has stuck, to my bemusement: He said that I look "like Superman's fitter grandfather."[2] In London there is even a group that has formed independently, made up of people who follow my philosophy. They had their first meeting in the fall of 2009 and get together regularly to discuss the program and swap stories about how it has changed their lives. There are now groups in New York City, Boston, and Houston.

I am very happy with my blog, which is available only to subscribers— and I plan to keep it that way. All the content is my own, expressed in my own way. No hype or miracles, just advice based on science and many years of experience.

CHAPTER 2

Before You Begin: Eight Things to Measure

Every diet and exercise plan tells you to consult with your doctor before you start, and this one is no different. But in addition to some tests performed as part of a standard annual checkup, I also recommend that you measure some things your physician might not typically check. A few of these measurements will simply be used as baseline numbers to help you determine just how much room for improvement you have; you might want to check them now and then check them again in six months to measure your progress. All of these measurements are important indicators of health and longevity. I depend on these benchmarks myself to assess how I'm doing.

1. Fasting Insulin Level

Your fasting insulin level is typically checked the morning after an overnight fast. It may be the single most important thing you can have tested. Fasting insulin is an indicator of your overall metabolic health, plain and simple. Insulin is so central to metabolism that it can accurately predict the outcomes of other tests that are commonly done.

Too-high insulin is associated with other worrisome values, such as high triglycerides, high blood pressure, low good (HDL) cholesterol, high bad (LDL) cholesterol, high C-reactive protein (CRP; a sign of inflammation), and elevated leptin (leptin and insulin work together, so when both are high, obesity is often present). Your insulin fasting level also will tell something about your internal fat deposits. A person with a large waistline and a high insulin level probably has sustained metabolic damage.

Among traditional Pacific Islander hunter-gatherers tested in what is known as the Kitava study, fasting insulin was found to be 5 international units per milliliter. In 2006, average fasting insulin in a sample of U.S. citizens was 11.4.

Physicians typically will not measure insulin levels unless they suspect a problem, so you may need to ask yours to prescribe this blood test for you.

2. Body Composition

Body fat isn't just extra weight you have to lug around; it also has a number of damaging effects on your health. It secretes hormones such as adiponectin, plasminogen activator inhibitor-1, and interleukin-6, which promote insulin resistance and harmful oxidation. When you carry excess fat, some of it travels throughout the body, ending up inside the liver, pericardium (the sac that holds the heart), and muscles. Fat also intrudes into other organs and tissues, disturbing their function. Fat is a source of inflammation; as fat cells die, they release their contents, and the immune system floods in to soak up the debris, resulting in inflammation.

Your body composition reflects your body's ratio of fat to muscle.[1] Body composition can be measured by the impedance method, which uses an electrical impulse to detect fat and muscle, or by a method called hydrostatic weighing, in which the entire body is submerged in water. This method relies on the fact that fat is lighter than muscle. The most common measurement used is the calipers test, which is less accurate than the other two but more practical. Using calipers, fat is measured at 7 to 12 sites on the body, and a body fat ratio is calculated. There are home scales that measure weight, body fat, and a variety of other things, but in my experience they are not terribly accurate.

Simply looking at yourself in a mirror reveals a great deal—nearly all you need to know. Many health authorities recommend a waist-to-hip ratio of about .95 for men and .88 for women, meaning a man's waist should be 95 percent as large as his hips; a woman's, 88 percent. But I believe that a better standard is approximately .8 for men and .7 for women—that's closer to the proportions of a modern athlete, and thus a close approximation to the proportions of early man.

There are two kinds of fat: visceral, which is found mostly in the belly and midsection; and subcutaneous, which lies just under the skin and is distributed more evenly throughout the body. Deep visceral fat pushes the gut out at the belly button. Someone with excessive visceral fat will have a robust look, because the fat doesn't sag, and his or her face will have some color to it. The color isn't an indication of ruddy good health but rather a sign of inflammation; the face will also be puffy. He or she will look somewhat husky, because metabolic syndrome causes fats and glycogen, a form of sugar, to build up in muscles, giving them a bigger look. Since he or she likely spends a lot of time sitting, an activity that promotes poor metabolism, someone with metabolic syndrome will have reduced muscle mass in the buttocks and legs—the pants will just hang.

Doctors say that apple-shaped obesity—where the fat is concentrated around the midsection—indicates a strong likelihood of cardiac disease. A waistline of more than 40 inches in men and more than 35 inches in women can itself be taken as a warning sign of impending heart trouble.[2]

Those with excessive subcutaneous fat will have flab that hangs over the belt, or a "muffin top" when squeezed into jeans. They will also typically have fat arms, hips, and thighs. This pear-shaped body is somewhat less prone to the metabolic syndrome, but all obesity is unhealthy.

Most doctors will weigh you, and then perhaps they will compute your body mass index (BMI), which is a number found by dividing your weight in kilograms by your height in meters squared. (You can spare yourself a lot of arithmetic by going online and finding one of the many instant BMI calculator Web sites; the National Institutes of Health provides one at http://www.nhlbisupport.com/bmi.)

Just to give you an idea of how this translates into reality according to BMI standards of health: A 5-foot-10 adult of either sex should weigh somewhere between 130 and 174 pounds. Anything under that is officially underweight; anything over that is overweight. Someone of that height weighing 209 pounds or more is considered to be obese. If you're 5-foot-5, you should, according to the BMI, weigh between 111 and 149 pounds. If you're under 111, you're considered underweight; if you're from 150 to 179, you're considered overweight; and if you're over 180, you're qualified as obese.

But you can have a "healthy" BMI according to the charts and still be too fat for optimum health. Or you may have a low weight because of too-little muscle tissue but still have too much fat. Such skinny-fat individuals look thin and may not be officially overweight. But with such poor body composition, they are at risk of diabetes. Older individuals tend to lose muscle and replace it with fat, meaning they are at risk of ill health even if the BMI number says otherwise. They may also lose weight from osteoporosis while becoming fatter.

Conversely, a lean, muscular person may have a high BMI. My BMI at 6-foot-1, 200 pounds is 26.4. According to the standard, I am overweight—a silly conclusion when you consider that my body is less than 8 percent fat. Because muscle weighs more than fat, most athletes fall into the overweight category by BMI standards. Generally speaking, the slightly overweight (BMI 25 to 30) fare better from a mortality point of view than the underweight (BMI under 18.5), obese (BMI over 30), or even normal (BMI 18.5 to 24.9), according to a 2005 study by Dr. Katherine Flegal published in the *Journal of the American Medical Association.*

3. Strength

Strength is a reliable predictor of mortality. The stronger you are, the longer you are likely to live. A physically strong, healthy body also decreases your chances of developing life-threatening diseases such as cancer, diabetes, or heart disease.

A person's life expectancy is a stair-step function of his or her strength; the strongest survive longer than the next strongest, and so on down the line. When testing is done and people are ranked according to strength, those in the top one-quarter live longer than those in the quarter below and even longer than those in each of the bottom two quarters. The chance of survival over the next 15 years is greatest in the top-ranked, strongest group; survival odds then decline for each lower strength group in a stair-step fashion. Cancer researcher Jonathan R. Ruiz and his coauthors tested more than 8,000 subjects age 20 to 82 for muscular strength.[3] They grouped individuals into three categories of strength and found that the age-adjusted risk of cancer was 17.5 per 10,000 in the weakest group, 11.0 in the middle group, and 10.3 in the strongest group. The weaker groups also had higher blood pressure, higher cholesterol, were more likely to have cardiovascular disease, and had a greater incidence of diabetes.

How strong should you be? As strong as you can get, because muscle is medicine against developing metabolic diseases. In effect, strength is a measure of your lean muscle mass, the primary site where your body disposes of glucose. Muscle is also your engine for life. The stronger you are, the more active you will be, simply because you expend less effort in everything you do. It may take all the power a weak person has to climb a flight of stairs, while a strong person can ascend with ease.

Strength may be tested in various ways. For example, a grip strength test is often used because it is convenient; there is a gripper device that some trainers and others use to measure strength. But it is less reliable than a test that involves a large muscle group, such as the legs or back. The leg press machine at your gym offers a reliable means of measurement because it involves many muscle groups and a large portion of the body's lean muscle mass. If, using two legs, you are able to press twice your weight, you would be in the strongest group in the Ruiz study population and have the lowest risk of cancer mortality. For me, that would require that I press 400 pounds, a challenge I can exceed with one leg.

4. Physiologic Capacity

Power is strength in action—the combination of speed and strength. Physiologic capacity—physical power—is a measure of your metabolic headroom, the space where your life occurs.

There are no standard tests for capacity, but more is always better. Thinking of physiologic capacity as your fight-or-flight capability suggests at least one good way to measure this. Football players are tested in the 40-yard or 100-yard dash. Your time in either one is a good measure of your ability to respond to a flight challenge. You can chart your progress accurately if you time your 40-yard dash once a month. You may at first have to walk the distance, then run it easily, then sprint lightly, building to a harder run as you progress. I can run the 40-yard dash in under 5 seconds. If my time rises above that level, I know that I am not doing the right things in the gym and that I ought to try a bit more sprinting. Of all athletes, those who sprint—basketball, soccer, and rugby players, as well as receivers, defensive backs, and running backs in football—are the most capable and have the best bodies.

Joggers are typically poor sprinters, and in my opinion, often have terrible bodies. Jogging is a useless exercise; as I will later explain, you are better off walking and mixing in a few playful sprints than jogging endlessly at a moderately taxing pace. For now, suffice it to say that no caveman ever jogged for miles while pursuing dinner or being chased by a predator. You either sprinted or starved, or were dinner yourself.

If you are so far gone that you hesitate to sprint, you have powerful evidence that your physiologic capacity is lousy. It seems that adults are reluctant to sprint, and so they miss the great benefits of this most important capacity. There is no good reason to lose this talent; it expresses our inner animal. It is a great mood lifter. Try it. Intermittent sprinting on a stationary bicycle (pedaling as fast as you can for 15-second bursts) is safer and easier than running in a field; you are less apt to step into a hole and injure yourself. I prefer to both run and bike.

I also suggest measuring physiologic capacity based on metabolic equivalent (MET), which is calculated as a multiple of your resting metabolic rate. A reading of 5 METs means you generated five times your resting metabolic rate. Children at play generate around 10 METs of peak power. The previously mentioned Ruiz study found that the maximal METs were 11.5 in the lowest strength category, 12.5 in the middle strength category, and 13.4 in the upper strength category. I can hit 30 METs, so I have a high physiologic capacity, more than twice the value of the highest group in the Ruiz sample of men, who are, on average, at least 30 years younger than me. Some cardio machines measure METs. While I don't recommend doing much cardio exercise, it can be helpful to use one of these machines occasionally to measure your capability.

5. Testosterone

This is an important hormone for males and females. Testosterone controls body composition for both sexes and is important for vitality. Low testosterone is associated with poor body composition, bad mood, depression, high blood pressure, low strength and energy, and metabolic syndrome. It could be used as a leading indicator of aging, since it begins to decline in most males after age 30. Overtraining and stress cause low testosterone. Marathoners have *very* low testosterone. My total testosterone of 660 nanograms per deciliter (just below the upper limit of the lab's scale, which goes from 350 to 720) is the highest my doctor has ever seen. Of course, most of the males he sees are overweight with high insulin, so this result is not so surprising.

There are no known supplements that will raise testosterone, because the level is tightly controlled in the body, but there are a few things that may help: Exercise, cut the booze, and drop the sugar.[4]

6. C-Reactive Protein

Your C-reactive protein level is among the most reliable predictors of cardiovascular inflammation and heart disease; as a result, most doctors will test for it. Research strongly supports the view that some heart disease is caused by inflammation, which itself is a by-product of obesity. CRP is a marker of inflammation and more accurately predicts cardiac events than triglycerides, cholesterol, or the ratio of either triglycerides or LDL cholesterol to HDL cholesterol. People with elevated CRP levels are at increased risk of diabetes, high blood pressure, and cardiovascular disease.[5] Obesity greatly raises the amount of CRP, because when the body has a large number of fat cells, the intrinsic rate of fat cell death increases—an obese person will have about three times as many fat cell deaths as a lean person. A dying fat cell prompts the immune system to clean up the debris; this means that an overweight person's immune system is being taxed more than that of someone weighing less. And inflammation also damages healthy tissues, such as the vascular lining.

The healthy reference range for CRP is zero to 2.13 milligrams per deciliter, and a healthy level is usually lower than 1. If hs-CRP level is lower than 1.0 mg/L, a person has a low risk of developing cardiovascular disease. If hs-CRP is between 1.0 and 3.0 mg/L, a person has an average risk. If hs-CRP is higher than 3.0 mg/L, a person is at high risk. My CRP is near the lower limit. This is a consequence of the low inflammatory burden of my diet and my low ratio of body fat to lean muscle mass. I suspect my intake of antioxidants through diet and supplements (which I will discuss later in this book) also helps to keep my CRP level low.

7. Good and Bad Cholesterol

Most doctors measure your cholesterol at your annual checkup. There are two cholesterol values you need to know: HDL and LDL. HDL is the "good" cholesterol. It gets its name from its ability to transport lipids back to the liver, where they can be metabolized. LDL is the "bad" cholesterol, the most readily oxidized form that creates lesions in the blood vessels.

My HDL level is 92, a value that exceeds the upper measurable range in some blood labs. My LDL level is just 98, which is below the no-risk level of 100.

The Wolfram Alpha science search engine measures the risk of heart disease based on data from the famous Framingham Heart study. You can go to the Web site (www.wolframalpha.com/input/ ?i=heart+attack+risk), input your cholesterol values and blood pressure, and come away with a good idea of your overall cardiac well-being.[6] When I enter my values (age 72, HDL 93, LDL 98, systolic blood pressure 120, diastolic blood pressure 70), I see that my 10-year risk of heart disease is a very low 5.7 percent, about equivalent to that of a 36-year-old male in good health. My wife's readings are similar to mine, but her risk profile was much higher before she began to eat as recommended in the New Evolution Diet. In spite of our ages, we should spend a long, healthy future together.

8. Triglycerides

Simply put, triglycerides are fats circulating in the bloodstream. Elevated triglycerides are almost always the result of metabolic disease. When insulin is chronically high and insulin resistance sets in, the body metabolizes glucose. Meanwhile, the fats just sit there in the bloodstream, where they are oxidized by free radicals, which are molecules that attack healthy cells. My triglyceride level is 49, near the bottom of the range. Your doctor should also measure the ratio of triglycerides to good cholesterol, which is another good predictor of cardiovascular disease. You can discuss the reference range with your doctor to assess your risk. My ratio, 0.53, is in the zero-risk range.

As I said at the start of this chapter, some of these tests must be ordered by a physician and carried out in the lab. Some of them may not be covered by your insurance, though most should be. Either way, the insight you'll gain into your current state of health and risk for future disease will be worth the effort and any extra expense.

CHAPTER 3

The New Evolution Diet

You want to eat smart. I want you to eat smart. So what does a smart diet look like?

A smart diet reduces the amount of energy (meaning food) you feel like consuming at the same time that it increases the amount of energy you feel like spending. And this occurs spontaneously, without any thoughts of cutting calories, or exercising more, or anything else. It just happens.

It improves the quality of your life by giving you more energy to expend on work, family, and play. It pleases the palette with beautiful food that is completely nutritious. It eliminates foods that interfere with your metabolism or set off your immune system. A smart diet relies on the millions of years of evolutionary design built into your appetite and metabolism to solve the problem of managing energy naturally, without a strict adherence to a plan.

The New Evolution Diet is a smart diet. It is relaxed, because it does not restrict calories—you eat all you want from a wide selection of fresh and nutritious foods that are delicious, aesthetically pleasing, and satisfying. It is not a top-down menu that requires you to restrict your calories or to follow directions and rigidly adhere to a schedule of meals and snacks. There are no rules. Rules are self-defeating, because nobody wants to be told what to eat or do—"That's why I became an adult," to borrow a line from Bob Newhart. A command-and-control diet creates stress. Stress encourages the release of cortisol, a hormone that promotes insulin resistance So stressing over diet and exercise is self-defeating—it actually makes you fatter.

It is nearly impossible to overeat on the New Evolution Diet because it is so complete and filling—it supplies the brain with all the energy and nutrients it needs while promoting a sensation of fullness in the stomach. That brain-stomach connection is important. When your brain is well nourished, it forgets about food. When your brain is improperly nourished, it becomes anxious and selfish and can think only about your next meal. Then you become lazy, because your brain curtails physical activity in order to protect its own energy supply. That means your body stops burning fat.

I want to emphasize this: A well-fed brain reduces your appetite and makes moving your body a pleasure. But when your brain is improperly nourished, it orders you to keep eating.[1]

Can you see how this dispels the hopelessly simple and damning explanation that is usually given for weight gain? You are not overweight because you eat too much and move too little. You eat too much and expend too little energy because you are overweight. Said another way, you are not what you eat; you are what your metabolism *does* with what you eat.

So we have to eat the right foods and avoid the wrong ones in order to keep the brain and body supplied with energy. Evolution designed your metabolism to perform that job, and it does so beautifully as long as you fuel it properly. Your metabolism wants you to have proper body composition. It doesn't care how many pounds you weigh. Believe it or not, that number will soon be irrelevant to you, too. It will become effortless for you to have a lean, beautiful, active body and a healthy, energetic brain.

Many fad diets encourage snacking throughout the course of the day. I think this is done to avoid scaring dieters away, but it's not a good idea. You should be eating enough in your regular meals to keep you satisfied. If you're not, you should adjust that rather than adding three daily mini-meals. The biggest problem with snacks is this: Every time you eat, you turn off your body's fat-burning mechanism. That's because your metabolism will always burn glucose before fat, and most snacks usually contain some glucose. So snacking actually thwarts your efforts to control weight. Eating between meals also keeps your insulin level higher than it needs to be.

I sometimes do snack, but only under certain circumstances. If I'm going to miss a meal, I will have a snack instead, maybe a slice of white-meat turkey. Or, before a meal, I may have a handful of nuts, some celery, or a pear—just to begin filling my belly and cutting my appetite.

In the early days of the diet, you may feel the need for an occasional snack. You should have one only if absolutely necessary, but make it fruit, vegetables, nuts, or lean meat—no carbs. Remember that if you just persevere and give your metabolism a chance to adjust to your new eating regime, you won't need to snack. The quality of your life should determine how much you eat. Instead of obsessing over how much you take in and then trying to burn it all off, you should focus on living a high-quality life and then eat to fulfill your energy demands. The pleasure and quality of life come from the energy you spend.

So what are you supposed to eat? In Chapter 5, I explain my eating habits as a way of suggesting some you might adopt. I am going to assume that you're not the kind of person who wants or needs someone to dictate to you exactly what to eat every day.

Here, as briefly as I can manage, is the New Evolution Diet.

In the United States, nutritional authorities at the U.S. Department of Agriculture (USDA) created and then refined, over the years, the familiar food pyramid, which groups foods into categories of varying sizes meant to suggest the essential components of a healthy diet. The USDA's five vegetable groups are dark green vegetables (such as broccoli, kale, spinach, and romaine lettuce); orange vegetables (various squashes, carrots, and sweet potatoes); dry beans and peas (black-eyed peas, lentils, kidney beans); starchy vegetables (corn, green peas, and potatoes); and other vegetables (artichokes, asparagus, bean sprouts, beets, brussels sprouts, cabbage, cauliflower, onions, tomatoes, zucchini, and so on). The other food groups in the USDA pyramid are grains, fruits, milk, meat and beans, and oils.

My diet eliminates many of these foods: dry beans and peas, starchy vegetables, grains, and dairy. Oils are restricted, with the exception of olive oil, and are primarily treated as spices or flavor enhancers. I add fresh spices as a category for their flavor and antioxidant value and add cheeses such as feta, romano, and Jarlsberg in sparing amounts strictly to add flavor to your meals.

One rationale for banishing grain-based foods—anything made with flour of any kind, or derived from corn or other grains—is that these did not exist when our genes stopped evolving, and so our bodies are not equipped to metabolize them. And there's an even better, more practical reason: Our dependence on simple carbohydrates and sugar as a means of sustenance has been one of the largest contributors to our current plagues of obesity and type 2 diabetes.[2] That includes rice, bread, pasta, and all baked goods. Having said that, I should add that I sometimes break my own commandment. I happen to love tacos, which contain both simple carbs *and* fats in the tortilla. I fill them with healthy ingredients such as fish and vegetables, but the fact remains that 40,000 years ago nobody ate tortillas. Which is fine—our goal is not to replicate exactly the paleo diet, just to learn from it. So I don't overdo it. I eat all the fish and vegetables but make sure to leave most of the tortilla.

My favorite dessert is cheesecake with a cup of great coffee. That breaks several of my commandments—the cake contains dairy, sugar, *and* simple carbs. I allow myself this treat maybe once a month—no more than that. I have eaten this way for so long that I don't feel deprived. But I wouldn't start this diet by breaking rules on a regular basis. By now, I have learned to love what this regimen permits, and my system reacts badly when I stray too far—I feel sluggish and stuffed when I eat foods like pizza or bread. My experience shows that it is better to cut out these foods altogether at first.

You've been led to believe that beans and legumes are healthy, I know, but in fact they are a mixed blessing. They contain plant proteins and other substances that cause a wide variety of ills that outweigh any benefits they may offer. Some legumes even contain toxins. I realize that advising you to stay away from beans is practically heresy. I'll explain my reasoning a little later in this chapter.

To replace the old food pyramid, I've devised one of my own. The shape conveys the general idea, but it cannot show the variation in food sources, which is a very important consideration. The water is a bit out of proportion, because you should not force yourself to drink. Simply rely on your thirst to indicate your body's needs. The brief exercise that most of us engage in presents no danger of dehydration. Leave the water bottle at home. It slows you down at the gym, and going a little thirsty now and then produces a hormone response that makes you better able to withstand actual thirst.

The New Evolution Diet Food Pyramid

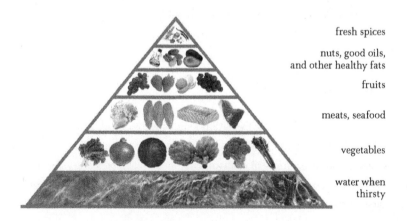

fresh spices

nuts, good oils, and other healthy fats

fruits

meats, seafood

vegetables

water when thirsty

Tenets of the New Evolution Diet

- Eat whole foods. These are foods that you (or someone else) can either pick or catch and kill.

- Eat at least some food raw. Try to have a salad or a piece of whole fruit once a day.

- Eat a wide variety of foods. This allows you to receive a larger array of nutrients. It also balances out the toxins you ingest. Everything you eat has toxins of one kind or another, even "natural" foods. Eating a wide variety of foods ensures that you don't get too much of any single toxin.

- Eat slowly and chew thoroughly. Your mom told you this.

- Do not eat many small meals during the course of the day. Give your body a chance to burn off excess fat by limiting yourself to two or three meals a day.

- Rule of thumb: Your diet should be one-third raw vegetables and fruit, one-third cooked vegetables, and one-third meat or fish. But remember, this is only a rough guide, not a decree.

- Do not deprive yourself of food. Even if dieting, you will make better progress when you are well nourished.

Vegetables

The first tier of the New Evolution Diet food pyramid, after water—which should be your drink of choice whenever you are thirsty—is vegetables. Choose a variety of colorful, low-starch vegetables every day and be sure to eat some raw. On the following page you'll find a list of vegetables I recommend eating regularly.

Vegetables to Eat

acorn squash	cauliflower	red peppers
artichokes	celery	romaine lettuce
asparagus	collard greens	spinach
bok choy	kale	tomatoes
broccoli	mushrooms	yams (in
brussels sprouts	mustard greens	moderation)
butternut squash	okra	zucchini
cabbage	onions	

Animal Protein

The next tier of the pyramid is animal protein—meat, fish, and eggs.

Research suggests you need to eat 1.5 grams of protein per kilogram of body weight daily. That comes to about 3 or 4 ounces of meat or fish in each meal, up to 15 ounces per day. If that feels like too much, you can reduce your meat and fish intake by taking a dietary supplement called branched-chain amino acids, which provides about 15 grams of amino acids per tablespoon.

Why is it so important to eat enough protein? Because your brain senses how much of it your body requires and prompts you to keep eating until you fulfill that need. This is why a diet lacking protein leads to obesity—your brain will always be telling you to eat more.[3] Eating meat and fish also promotes a feeling of fullness, or satiety. Adequate protein intake is essential to maintaining bone mass. This is why it is especially important for women, who tend to lose more bone mass than men as they age, to get enough protein in their diet. Insufficient tryptophan and excessive carbohydrate intake may also

Protein to Eat

MEAT	POULTRY	SEAFOOD
game meats	chicken	anchovies
ham	duck	bass
lamb	turkey	cod
lean beef		herring
liver		mackerel
pork		salmon
veal		sardines
		shellfish
		snapper
		squid

contribute to a deficiency in the neurotransmitter serotonin, a likely factor in depression.

Organic, grass-fed meat is preferable, as is free-range poultry. Red meat is fine, in moderation, but (white-meat) poultry is generally healthier. You should aim to eat a variety of meats and seafood, and roughly equal amounts of each. Above is a list of healthy options.

Larger fish (such as tuna, king mackerel, swordfish, shark, and tilefish) should be eaten sparingly, because they can contain higher concentrations of mercury from the smaller fish they eat. Game can be difficult to find unless you hunt it yourself. But game meats are a good, low-fat source of protein and don't contain the chemicals, hormones, and antibiotics sometimes found in commercially raised meat. Game birds include duck, goose, quail, squab, and pheasant. Game meats include bison, rabbit, venison, and boar. Boar sausage is one of my favorites.

Fruit

The third tier of the pyramid is fruit. Fruit offers antioxidants and many other plant compounds that are beneficial to your health. But do go easy on fruit consumption. Pay attention to portion size, as some modern fruits are bred to contain extra sugar. (Those huge strawberries you see at the supermarket, for instance, contain a great deal of it.)

Fruits to Eat

apples	lemons	pineapple
avocado	limes	plums
blueberries	mangoes	raspberries
cantaloupe	oranges	strawberries
cherries	papaya	watermelon
honeydew melons	pears	
grapes, especially dark red ones		

Four or five servings of fruit a day is plenty; more than that and you're getting a lot of fructose, which is just another form of sugar. Melons are great; watermelon is excellent, since it contains the antioxidant glutathione and its precursors. It may also elevate testosterone, which, as I mentioned earlier, is necessary for good health in both men and women. Avoid bananas (which have too much carbohydrate), dried fruits, and all fruit juice and canned fruits.

Nuts and Good Oils

Nuts, oils, and other healthy fats comprise the fourth tier of the food pyramid. Nuts should be eaten in moderation. You'll notice that my list does *not* include cashews, which are toxic to eat raw; "raw" cashews are actually processed, though not roasted, and are high in carbohydrates. Neither should you eat peanuts, which are actually legumes, not nuts. Stay away from seeds, too, which are loaded with toxins and *anti*nutrients. Below are the nuts I recommend eating, in order of healthiness.

Nuts to Eat

almonds   walnuts   pecans

most of the others (brazil nuts, filberts, so on)

The term "good oils" is somewhat of a misnomer, because the truth is that no oil is particularly *good* for you. I know that olive oil has been described as a healthy food, and in fact it is the only oil I eat. I use it on salads and, in very small quantities, in cooking, mainly for the flavor it imparts. But it doesn't really do much to improve your health, except that it is less bad than all the other oils people use. Remember, we consumed no vegetable-based oils at all even as recently as 200 years ago. If you do cook with olive oil, never allow it to get so hot that it smokes—if it reaches that temperature, it is being oxidized, and free radicals are being formed.

Good Oils to Eat

olive oil   omega-3 fish oil (supplement)   castor oil

Beyond that, I take an omega-3 fish oil supplement on days when I don't eat fish. There is abundant evidence that omega-3 oils have a beneficial effect on inflammation and even obesity. The docosahexaenoic acid (DHA) and eicosapentaenoic acid (EPA) content of fish oil also promotes brain health. Sometimes I take a cod liver oil capsule instead, for the omega-3 oils and vitamins A and D it contains.

But most common kitchen oils—canola, vegetable, corn, palm—are unnecessary. If you must cook in oil and want to do so at a higher temperature than permitted by olive oil, then use canola oil (made from rapeseed but called "canola" because it is a more felicitous name). By now most people know to avoid any hydrogenated oils and products that contain them (such as margarine), because they produce trans fats, which are harmful and completely alien to our bodies.

Foods to Not Eat

Some of the most frequently asked questions I receive about the New Evolution Diet begin "Why can't I eat . . . ?" Here are some common foods to avoid—and why you should avoid them.

Grains

Oh, yes—it's that dietary staple that the USDA esteems so highly. But simply stated, our bodies are not genetically adapted to process grains. Grains cause allergic reactions, high insulin levels, obesity, and digestive disorders. Remember that this also includes corn—which is a grain, not a vegetable.

Keep in mind that grains are simply seeds of grass. They contain many antinutrients whose job is to damage or limit the reproduction capabilities of the herbivorous creatures, bacteria, and fungi that consume them. The seeds of plants don't have fight-or-flight powers; their sole means of protection are these toxins and antinutrients. The seeds of apples and apricots contain arsenic; the castor bean contains ricin, one of the most powerful toxins; soybeans contain plant estrogens that, if eaten in large quantities, may limit the ability of male herbivores to reproduce and may promote early maturation among young women and heighten the risk of breast cancer; and wheat contains glutens that can damage the gut of herbivores (and humans, especially for people who suffer from celiac disease). One of the most striking examples of the sophisticated defense system evolved by plants is a protein in the tamarisk tree that alters gene expression in locusts in such a way that the flight muscles of the larvae fail to develop.

Another good reason to give up grains is the fact that they contain a group of plant proteins called lectins. Consumption of lectins has been linked to leptin resistance in the body. Leptins are hormones that regulate appetite, energy, metabolism, and reproduction. The leptin gene is highly conserved across different species; it is thought to have evolved in primates some four to seven million years ago. Leptin tells your body when you've had enough to eat—as with insulin resistance, leptin resistance itself is a cause of obesity. Given the exalted PR that bread gets in the Bible (among other places), it's hard to demonize it, I realize. Just remember that your genes were born many millennia before the biblical era and therefore remain unimpressed. Bread is the ultimate poverty food—it exists only because grain is cheap, easy to grow, and virtually imperishable. Now, in the age of domesticated protein and refrigeration, bread has outlived its usefulness. It is an inferior food that has no place in a healthy diet. The same is true of anything made with flour (pasta, baked goods) or other grains (rice, barley, corn). It's fine for herbivorous animals. Not for you.

Eating whole grains is slightly healthier than eating the refined variety. But it's not as good as simply avoiding them altogether.

Dairy

You may eat some dairy, such as unsweetened yogurt or cheese in small amounts. Always choose organic dairy products from grass-fed cows.

Humans are genetically adapted to mother's milk until weaning. We are the only animal that drinks milk into adulthood and consumes another creature's milk. Processed cow's milk contains excess growth hormones such as recombinant bovine growth hormone (rBGH) and insulin-like growth factor (IGF-1). (Calves, unlike you, have to grow a lot in a hurry.) Milk and beef products have certain levels of naturally-occurring trans fats. Commercially raised dairy cattle live in unsanitary conditions and are exposed to high levels of bacteria. They are routinely injected with antibiotics, and some of these antibiotics find their way into the milk stocked in the grocery store. The proteins in cow's milk may also trigger an immune response and promote insulin resistance in humans.

Starchy Foods

This category includes potatoes, which are not vegetables, technically speaking, but tubers—plant forms that specialize in storing energy. It also includes most root vegetables, such as sweet potatoes, parsnips, water chestnuts, turnips, and radishes. A yam (which is different from a sweet potato) every now and then is fine because it contains a lot of fiber, which slows the release of the starches. The occasional beet or raw carrot is fine, too. Other starchy vegetables to avoid include green beans and lima beans.

Oils and Fats

This category includes all oils except for olive and canola, mentioned earlier, and maybe a little sesame oil for taste. It goes without saying that butter and lard should be avoided completely. You'll get the fats your body needs from the animal protein you eat and healthy fats from plant sources, such as avocados.

Salt

Salt itself is essential and not a toxin. But the level at which we currently consume it is extravagant; average daily intake is around 3,375 milligrams, whereas it was probably less than 700 milligrams during the Paleolithic period. While the kidneys of a healthy individual might be able to handle this overload, many people now develop hypertension because of a defect in their ability to clear that much sodium. People get most of their salt not from the shaker but from processed foods and drinks. By avoiding these foods, the New Evolution Diet keeps salt at a low, healthy level. I use no salt beyond what is naturally in my foods.

Nonfoods

By now this should be a no-brainer. Just because you can eat it doesn't mean that it's food. This includes all those processed goodies like chips, doughnuts, snack cakes, baked goods, candy, and ice cream. *"What about on my birthday?"* you ask? Well, how about living to celebrate many more, I answer. Oh, I suppose a little cake once a year would be okay. Even I eat a bit of cheesecake every once in a while. Personally, though, I would rather have a delicious lobster dinner to celebrate *my* birthday.

Certain Plant-Based Foods

Somehow, we have all absorbed the idea that anything that grows in the earth must be healthy to eat. While it's true that most fruits and vegetables are good for us and should be a major part of our diet, there are also plants that promote obesity and make us sick. It's not as though plants *want* us to eat them. They don't really care whether or not you're in good health.

Plants that did not protect themselves from pathogens did not survive. So, when we eat a potato, we ingest its protective toxins. Or, we may trigger a plant's evolutionary defense against an herbivore, which by eating the plant voraciously limits its reproduction.

Soy and soy products (including soy sauce, tofu, textured vegetable protein, soy milk, and edamame) should be avoided because soy is high in lectins and estrogen. In its natural state, the soybean is not edible. It must be processed at high temperatures to remove toxins.

Peanuts—which are legumes, not nuts—are another food to avoid. They contain one of the most carcinogenic toxins known: aflatoxin. Peanuts get this toxin from the soil in which they grow, and it often breeds when peanuts are stored improperly and become moldy. Peanut (and soy) allergies are occasionally fatal. All podlike foods, which include beans, lentils, and legumes, are actually seeds of one form or another. If seeds were too tasty and nutritious, the plant world would never have survived this long. There is an evolutionary arms race fought between plants and the animals that eat them. A highly nutritious plant that did not defend itself or its seeds would become extinct. By eliminating grains, beans, legumes, and milk from your diet, you will shift the pH balance of your food and therefore your body from acidic toward a more neutral and even slightly alkaline state. You will also remove the phytic acids that interfere with mineral metabolism. This is a very good thing. It will permit better mineral metabolism, adding density to your skeletal mass. This is especially important for children's diets. Grains were a major factor in the rickets epidemic that plagued Great Britain at the turn of the 20th century, causing developmental problems that included stunted growth, bowed legs, a sunken nasal and upper jaw area of the face, bad teeth, and clubbed feet. During the Industrial Revolution, poor children were fed an all-grain diet deficient in calcium, zinc, and protein and suffered as a result.

In our modern times, consuming too many grain-based carbs, too much coffee, and too many soft drinks (which contain phosphoric acid) seems to contribute to our eventual loss of bone mass. All these products induce an acidic condition that the body buffers by using bone calcium as an antacid.

You can tell the New Evolution Diet is guided by a relatively low-carb philosophy, although not as much as some other diets. Many people mistakenly believe low-carb eating is a "fad." But eating this way has proven to be healthy, and it was an important part of our evolution as a species. To call a diet on which humans lived for millennia a fad is just ignorance. In fact, it is the modern fad of eating a high-carb, high-grain, high-sugar diet that is harmful.

Why Our Ancestors Were Not Vegetarians

From time to time I am asked, "Can you be a vegetarian on the New Evolution Diet?" The short answer is yes, as long as you get adequate protein and other essential nutrients. But my question for you is this: *Why* would you want to be a vegetarian? Unless you choose to abstain from eating meat because you value the lives of animals, or because commercial livestock farming takes an undue toll on the environment, I think you should reconsider.

Just a few millennia ago, it would have been impossible to survive as a vegetarian. Wild plants would have been an insufficient source of nourishment. The last vegetarian human precursors did not endure. Their brains could not develop, because they didn't get enough fatty acids and protein through their diet. They had to eat all day just to stay nourished, and so they had large stomachs, small brains, and little mobility. They were rather like gorillas—vegetarian primates.

Dental isotopes of Neanderthals show them to be just below the wolf in their carnivory; they passed from the scene about 35,000 years ago. But Cro-Magnon (*Homo sapiens*) dentition reveals that they were only slightly less carnivorous. And they are the predecessors to us all. In *Nutrition and Evolution,* Michael Crawford and David Marsh argue that the human brain requires more fatty acids (EPA and DHA in particular) than can be produced by consuming plants alone.[1]

Only in a world with a safe and vast supply of food can one even consider vegetarianism as an option. But even then it is not an easy choice. A vegetarian diet forces excess reliance on high-carbohydrate, high-glycemic foods. There is no other way to obtain adequate calories. Otherwise, you have to eat so frequently and so much that you can't be very active.

The few vegetarian students I knew at the University of California, Irvine, seemed to think a potato chip was a vegetable. They ate so poorly that I don't know how they made it through school. Children raised without eating animal protein will have underdeveloped nervous systems and brains. Many vegetarians I know are technically not overweight, but they have terrible body composition—they have too little lean body mass and too much fat, and they look stressed and puffy. They're skinny-fat.

Populations in countries like India, Iraq, and Egypt, where vegetarianism is widely practiced, are experiencing a sharp rise in the number of new cases of type 2 diabetes. There are many theories that attempt to explain this phenomenon, from increased migration to urban centers to the influence and availability of Western foods, but I believe this rate can be attributed to the consumption of large amounts of rice and other simple, high-glycemic foods that damage the metabolism and promote insulin resistance, thus accelerating aging and the development of diabetes.

If you want to remain a vegetarian, I suggest that you take adequate vitamin B complex and fat-soluble vitamins such as A. You will also benefit from taking a branched-chain amino acid complex, one with little or no sugar or near-sugars. The leucine in the complex will encourage protein synthesis. And get adequate fats from olive and omega-3 oils. Most vegetables available to us today are not as nutritious as those our ancestors consumed. I eat a lot of meat. Carnivores can love the environment, too. Open-range animals are raised on clean rangeland, which preserves open space. They eat a variety of plants and insects and have little body fat or saturated fat. For that reason, game is excellent food. My favorite restaurant here in Utah is Buffalo Bistro in the little town of Glendale, along Highway 89 on the way to Bryce Canyon National Park. Its boar sausage and buffalo steaks are the greatest.

CHAPTER 4

How to Not Eat

Just as we must learn to eat properly, we should also learn how to *not* eat. For a variety of reasons, none having to do with counting calories, I recommend that you undertake the occasional mini-fast. Once a week or so, you should eat little, skip dinner, or eat nothing at all for a day.

I'm not suggesting you starve yourself: If you go hungry today, you should make up for it tomorrow by eating a bit more. I realize that the idea of skipping a meal or going a day without food is unsettling to most people. One of my blog readers told me that it was the most frightening part of this plan. Having gone on to lose some 70 pounds and replace his fat with lean muscle, he has since become a dedicated advocate of intermittent fasting.

Every living creature since the beginning of time has gone hungry now and then. Intermittent fasting is imbedded in our metabolism; food scarcity was a normal part of life for our ancestors. The research suggests that prehistoric hunter-gatherers spent about one-third of their lives hungry, which is more deprivation than we need for our purposes. But a little self-imposed food scarcity is a good thing.[1]

In fact, our bodies respond to it in an interesting way: Brief fasting improves insulin sensitivity and protein turnover in muscle.

A little hunger turns on your body's repair mechanisms. So doing without the occasional feeding is a powerful way to slow aging. I skip one dinner a week, chosen at random. On those nights, I go to bed early. You burn fat while you sleep. The more sleep you get, the leaner you will be.

You may already be aware of the scientific research into calorie restriction (CR) as a way of extending life and promoting better health. The practice has become a small but impassioned global movement. Advocates of calorie restriction suggest that you subsist on 900 to 1,000 calories a day instead of our typical 2,000 to 2,500 calories. Some studies conducted in animals and other organisms support this theory. Calorie restriction has been shown to improve health markers in rats, primates, and humans. It may extend life span, at least in yeast, worms, and flies.[2]

Because reduced calorie intake lowers the metabolic rate, CR stabilizes your body's cell membranes by reducing their rate of damaging oxidation and their polyunsaturated fat content. The higher the polyunsaturated fat content of the membrane, the shorter the life span in mammals. (This surprising news should be a little unsettling to the omega-3 crowd, myself included. I try to balance the polyunsaturated fat content of my cell membranes through periodic fasting and the use of antioxidants. But you can't control everything.)

Here is where I part with the believers in chronic dietary restriction: Aside from the chronic misery of living on so little food, CR can have a negative impact on health. Your body's stress response itself becomes a problem. CR diets affect the brain, which may lose cortical mass with prolonged food deprivation. Studies have shown that those who completely deprive themselves of food—anorexics—have shriveled brains, which may be an underlying reason for their inability to recover from their dangerous behavior.[3] The type of intermittent fasting I suggest actually protects the brain by increasing its sensitivity to insulin, which reduces both inflammation and oxidation. Chronic CR, unless practiced with high sophistication, may not.

While most of the research that's been conducted on CR has explored the antiaging benefits of chronic food deprivation, it is becoming clear that intermittent caloric deprivation may be equally effective. Mild intermittent stressors like fasting and exercise can be enough to increase resistance to disease and improve or extend quality of life. Eating half your normal intake one day and then one and a half times your normal diet the next is as beneficial as restricting calories every day.[4]

Intermittent fasting has been shown to increase the average and maximum life span by as much as 67 percent in rodents.[5] It has also been found to decrease the incidence of tumors and kidney disease in animals, and it may potentially be a useful practice (the studies on this are not yet definitive) for stroke patients and those with Alzheimer's, Parkinson's, and Huntington's diseases, as it may help to increase the body's resistance to dysfunction and degeneration. Intermittent fasting enhances resistance to oxidative, metabolic, and other types of stress. It is nice to know that our obsession with eating regularly is so wrong. Go ahead and skip that meal, and reap the rewards of better metabolism and enhanced resistance to stress and disease.

The benefits of calorie restriction, we are learning, come primarily from the restriction of glucose in the diet. So, just by eating the diet I recommend, you can achieve the same benefits as CR bestows. And you won't have to go hungry and cranky for the rest of your life.[6]

Experiments with bacteria show that life extension for these one-celled organisms can be gained by switching their fuel from glucose to fat, or by shutting down chronic sugar burning through exercise, which burns out the glycogen in the cell.[7] (Yes, scientists can even make bacteria exercise.) Unfortunately, so far all the research is being done on microbes. I hope they get around to studying it in humans soon.

Here's how cutting out glucose works on your cells. The genes that control aging and life span do so by using what is known as the insulin-IGF (insulin-growth factor) pathway. We're all familiar by now with insulin, the hormone made in the pancreas whose job it is to make nutrients in the blood available to the body. Less known is IGF-1, a potent anabolic hormone manufactured primarily in the liver that increases cellular metabolism, enhances the function of tissues, and participates in glucose homeostasis, which maintains blood glucose within a healthy range. Together, insulin and IGF control growth and glucose metabolism in humans and other organisms. The economic feedback loop between glucose and life span likely exists in all organisms; insulin-IGF-1 signaling exists in everything from worms to humans.

That connection was critical to humans 40,000 years ago, when carbohydrate was a rare nutrient. Glucose—the by-product of carbohydrates—became a valuable internal signal conveying information about our environment. A low glucose flow through the brain's detection circuits would be a clear signal of scarcity; a high flow would be a signal of abundance and a sign that the body should store some of that surplus energy in the form of fat.

The hypothalamus is a brain region that produces the hormones that regulate food intake and energy metabolism. Rats with decreased levels of insulin receptors in the hypothalamus eat voraciously and are insulin-resistant in other tissues as well. This suggests that insulin signaling in the brain can regulate body weight and energy metabolism in a way that is consistent with the aging effect of insulin-IGF-1 signaling.

"Diabetes of the brain," as insulin resistance is sometimes called, contributes to unhealthy, accelerated aging. It promotes overeating, poor glucose control, and oxidation of brain cells. I have often wondered why some type 2 diabetics I know are so apt to overeat; their hunger is often voracious, even though they store thousands of calories of energy in their fat. They eat as though they have brain damage, and in fact, some or all of them probably do have damaged brains. The inflammation produced by their elevated blood glucose damages the energy-sensing circuits of the brain. Brain imaging shows that the obese have shrunken brains.[8] Diabetes of the body may promote diabetes of the brain. And the areas of the brain most vulnerable are those that are associated with the development of Alzheimer's disease.

As noted, glucose restriction may protect the body and the brain by turning down the insulin-IGF-1 signaling pathway. The signal of glucose abundance is also tied to DNA expression. During times of plentiful nutrition, the most effective way for DNA to propagate itself is through reproduction, since there is enough energy to support offspring. When there is no excess glucose, DNA is best served by not reproducing. Low levels of insulin and carbohydrate are what send that signal, in which case it is in the DNA's interest to preserve itself for as long as possible through gene repair, stress resistance, and cell maintenance. For DNA to self-propagate most efficiently, it has evolved this simple and economic feedback loop.

The existence of this feedback seems to be well established and suggests a number of ways to improve health in humans. (See the research cited in the notes for Chapters 4 through 9.) The message of glucose scarcity is what we want to send to our bodies, even if a little trickery is required. We want our DNA to focus on gene repair and stress resistance.[9]

I choose to live like a wild human rather than a lab rat. I opt for intermittent, ad hoc calorie restriction, retaining my lean body mass while enjoying, as far as I can see, the full benefits of CR.[10] I also exercise and, thus, expose my body to another form of CR—an acute negative energy balance. In most things, the wild human is my role model. We would all do better if we relearned how to be good animals.

CHAPTER 5

A Month on the New Evolution Diet

Some New Evolution Diet followers tell me they have a bit of trouble in the beginning. Meaning: They have a difficult time abandoning the idea that they must cut calories and exercise more if they want to lose weight.

When I tell them they ought to focus on making muscle instead of dropping pounds, they begin to understand.

The New Evolution Diet is intended to alter your metabolism to favor muscle and brain tissue over fat. Once people see that proper eating and exercise can achieve that goal, the program begins to make sense. They learn to focus on body composition—the balance of muscle versus fat—instead of calories or weight, and they give up the idea that they have to starve in order to lose pounds.

I have a lot of muscle mass, a little over 80 kilograms' worth, which is roughly double that of the average man my age. Our lean body mass burns calories even when we are idle—every 22 pounds of it burns about 100 calories a day. I burn 300 to 365 more calories every day than the average person my age even when doing nothing (something I do quite a lot).[1]

I also expend more energy when I play or exercise, and my superior state of health permits me to be more active throughout the day than most people my age.

I eat heartily and never gain weight. For example, here's what a typical day's diet looks like for me:

Breakfast: half a ham steak cooked in a pan, three hard-boiled egg whites, and half a cantaloupe

Lunch: a huge salad of romaine lettuce, raw broccoli, cauliflower, red cabbage, kalamata olives, half an avocado, and about 9 ounces of smoked salmon, dressed with balsamic vinegar and olive oil

Dinner: half a rack of barbecued baby back ribs, asparagus sautéed in garlic and olive oil, and half a red pepper grilled with the ribs

Not exactly starvation.

The people who have the most difficulty adjusting to the New Evolution Diet are usually those who had the unhealthiest diets beforehand. Some people continue to experience serious sugar cravings. To them, I recommend taking a tablespoon of a branched-chain amino acid supplement, which is available at most health food stores. It will decrease your craving for sweets because your liver will convert amino acids to the amount of glucose your body needs (but no more)[2]. Eating a piece of fruit may deter sugar cravings, but the main problem with any diet that restricts what you eat is compliance. Most dieters cheat. They do so because they are hungry and their brains suddenly have to manage with less glucose from food sources. And as I mentioned earlier, a brain that lacks glucose has no willpower. In other words, a traditional diet makes it harder for you to resist carbs and sugar, not easier.

The other problem is monotony. Most diets require too much regimentation, too much work and thought. They bore you. This is not an issue on the New Evolution Diet, because you can eat a wide array of delicious, satisfying food without worrying about planning meals or counting calories. There is no routine or boredom, because variation and randomness are part of the strategy.

Some of my online followers have been practicing this diet for a decade or more. People write to me to share their stories and celebrate their success. One man wrote,

> The biggest change is in my cravings and mood swings. I never feel cranky before a meal or sleepy after. Several of my family members are on board and have had similar success. This has literally changed my life.

A 35-year-old woman who previously had been intimidated by the New Evolution Diet philosophy wrote,

> Once I started, I was surprised how easy it was. I dropped 6 pounds in the first week (for a total of 9 so far, with my body continuing to tighten even without a change on the scale). Immediately, I noticed that my ankles didn't get puffy and swell anymore in the heat. I found myself standing up straighter without effort, and sitting upright in my chair at work. My skin looked different—bright, tight, and glowing. Without changing anything else, I suddenly had enormous amounts of stamina. I felt like a superhero—and decided sugar and flour were my kryptonite.
>
> Perhaps most important to me, my mood changed significantly. I used to be prone to flashes of anger or sadness, and while I am generally a calm person, I would often lose my temper or my cool if things went wrong. I became a calmer, wiser, more responsive version of myself. Instead of panicking and reacting, I'm now able to coolly survey the facts and make a smart decision. I know without a doubt this has led to a series of promotions at work—my calm was taken as evidence of leadership.
>
> Oh, and while I've always looked young for my age, I'm now told that I look younger than both my sisters—including one who is 8 years younger than I am. In fact, I was carded for a drink

recently and the waitress was genuinely surprised. "I hope *I* look that good at 35," she said.

By the end of the first week on the New Evolution Diet, you will probably have lost about 5 pounds. You will appear less puffy and the pinkness in your face will diminish—these are signs that you are less inflamed. You should be sleeping better, as well as burning plenty of fat as you sleep, and feeling less fatigued.

As mentioned in the stories above, many people also experience a brightening of mood. That's because the energy and nutrients meant for your brain will no longer be siphoned off by your fat. Your hormones will stop releasing a big burst of insulin after you eat, a response that sends blood glucose crashing an hour later. Your brain's reaction to that glucose crash is to release stress hormones, which raise blood pressure and elevate feelings of anxiety.

I have come to the conclusion that many people develop a conditioned fear of starvation through those repeated glucose crashes. That causes the release of more stress hormones, which only increase the intensity of the crash. When the stress hormone cortisol and insulin combine, they overwhelm any so-called willpower you might possess and make it nearly impossible to resist the urge to eat fat and sugar. Your cravings are not a sign of psychological weakness—they have physiological origins.[3]

As you will see, it really is easy to begin this eating plan. In the following pages, I've listed what a typical four weeks might look like for you on the New Evolution Diet. These suggestions are based on my own diet and exercise regimen. While you don't have to eat exactly like I do, hopefully looking at a typical month for me will inspire you to create your own routine. There are just a few things to master, and you will learn to do so in the first week.

Start by writing down all the appalling things you have been eating. I won't list examples of them here—you know what they are. Note especially how many grams of carbohydrates you usually take in. Keep the list as a reminder of how far offtrack one can get through habit and lack of consideration. Now you're ready to begin fueling your body the right way.

Week 1

Monday

BREAKFAST
Have some salmon—smoked, canned, or fresh—and pair it with a salad or celery and melon. Celery is a great source of fiber. Melon is a good source of minerals and antioxidants.

LUNCH
Make a big fresh salad full of vegetables such as broccoli, cabbage, green onions, and artichoke hearts or hearts of palm. Top it with steamed shrimp, roast turkey, or grilled chicken and add half a chopped avocado. Use olive oil with balsamic vinegar as a dressing.

DINNER
Grill some barbecued beef or pork ribs. Add a big helping of asparagus and a romaine salad. Eat no later than 7 P.M. If you can't eat before then, have a snack instead of a meal—a few slices of lean turkey breast with half a sliced avocado. Have a handful of nuts if you still don't feel satisfied.

EXERCISE
Learn the abdominal brace. Stand tall and bend slightly forward from the hips as you feel the erector muscles tighten in your lower back. Hold them flexed and stand straight. Then, holding that position, push

your stomach out a bit. Then lift your heart and look out over your cheekbones as you walk without tilting your head down. This is a position of power that protects and strengthens the spine and lets you see the world in a different way.

Tuesday

BREAKFAST

Make an omelet (two eggs, one yolk) with well-cooked and drained bacon, fresh fruit, and black coffee. Drink water as needed.

LUNCH

Italian, but how can you eat Italian without carbs? I did it for 2 weeks in Italy just by passing on the bread and pasta, the *primi piatti.* Send the bread back, and order a salad and a fish or seafood entrée with vegetables. Drink fresh water with lemon and have a cup of espresso, plain with no sugar or cream.

DINNER

Grill a flank steak or rump steak. This is a very lean cut of beef and contains ample protein. I marinate mine in a small amount of low-sodium teriyaki sauce that I buy at the supermarket. We are not trying to literally live in the Ice Age, just to emulate aspects of that diet, taking our tastes and what is available in stores into account. Just sear a lean flank or rump steak on both sides and cook it medium rare. Cut up some squash and red peppers, splash on some olive oil, and put them on the grill with the steak. A glass of wine right about now would be great, but in the first month you should cut out all alcohol. Your liver will love you for it, and if you have been eating the way most people do, you have some fat accumulating there.[4]

EXERCISE

Establish your balance in bare feet. Stand tall; settle the weight into your hips and into your feet just before the heels. Lift one foot and shift your weight to the other. Notice how much you sway. Maintain balance on the ball and heel of the foot and by flexing your hip muscles. Good balance can be learned and makes you move gracefully and safely. Your posture and movement can take years off your appearance. Learn to stand and walk like you are proud of your body.

Wednesday

BREAKFAST
Have a couple of pieces of Canadian bacon or ham with two hard-boiled egg whites and some cantaloupe with coffee and plenty of water. Let your hunger determine the size of your portions. Eat all you want but no more.

LUNCH
Order two grilled fish tacos with cabbage, pico de gallo, and fresh salsa, with water or unsweetened iced tea. Don't worry about the tortilla—eat as much of it as you need to get the fish and cabbage into your mouth and leave the rest. Or, forget the tortilla and eat with a fork. No rice or beans.

DINNER
How hungry are you right now, truly? At night I often eat only a salad with smoked salmon, red cabbage, garlic, celery, kalamata olives, and avocado. I add a smoked anchovy or two. The bulk will fill you, and the nutrition is excellent. You can use any canned seafood you like; canned crab is OK but fresh is even better for you.

EXERCISE
Start your day with a walk in the briskness of the morning and enjoy the chill. Don't wear a jacket, just dress lightly in a shirt and shorts if possible. Your metabolism will thank you, and your "brown fat," or

adipose, tissues will fire up. If you feel up to it, sprint lightly a couple of times during your walk.

Thursday

BREAKFAST

Make four hard-boiled eggs, but don't eat two of the yolks. Eggs are healthy, but you should skip the yolks now and then. The yolk is mostly fat (that's what the hatching chick eats), while the white is mostly protein. Eat some fresh fruit of your choice.

LUNCH

If you have time, take a walk for lunch and along the way find a sandwich shop that has good pastrami. Ask for the meat only, without the bread. Have unsweetened iced tea or water to drink, but drink plenty of it, since the pastrami is salty. After you eat, continue strolling. It is a walk interrupted by food, not really a break; but neither is it a "power" walk or a rushed one. The walk is to relax, to look around at the people and scenery, and to plan your afternoon.

DINNER

You will be hungry if you are like me. It is time for a grilled swordfish steak or orange roughy with a great vegetable salad.

EXERCISE

At work, climb a flight of stairs; drive your movement from the hip and raise your foot high as you climb. Stand when you take phone calls. Your call will be shorter and more to the point. Do some sprinting when you get home from work before supper. Or play football in the backyard with your children. A bit of exercise before eating increases insulin sensitivity.

Friday

Friday can be a busy, stressful day. You handle stress better if you eat less, and maybe you're planning a dinner out with friends or family. So have a light breakfast of nuts and fruit. Almonds, walnuts, or mixed nuts are preferred. If they're salted, it should be with sea salt, and lightly at that.

BREAKFAST

Look in your refrigerator and find some leftover dinner or lunch to eat. If you have no leftovers, brown two pork chops in their own fat with some fresh rosemary and eat them with a bit of cantaloupe.

LUNCH

I suggest a salad of vegetables, lettuce, plenty of celery, and some lean chicken or seafood.

DINNER

Your options are wide open—just make good choices. Send the bread back, kill the croutons, and select your meal wisely from vegetables, seafood, and lean meat. Try not to eat carbohydrates with fat. That means skipping the potatoes and gravy and the pasta with cheese.

EXERCISE

Try working on your balance and your posture in the morning or at work for a break. For activity, practice walking in the office, campus, or warehouse—wherever you work—with your new posture while doing the abdominal brace. Lift your heart and look over your cheekbones as you walk. I bet you'll get some compliments.

Saturday

BREAKFAST
Find some leftovers from earlier this week—meats and seafood make the best, quickest breakfasts. If you don't have any leftovers, make a dozen hard-boiled eggs for the week. Eat some hard-boiled egg whites and a few pieces of some lean turkey breast.

LUNCH
Make or buy a salad with lean protein, such as smoked salmon or fresh grilled tuna, and vegetables like red cabbage, broccoli, tomato, cauliflower, celery, kalamata olives, fresh garlic, and spring onions. You can use olive oil and balsamic vinegar for dressing and fresh herbs for seasoning.

DINNER
I would have steak covered with grilled shrimp in a garlic and lemon sauce along with sautéed asparagus and grilled banana squash. Cut the squash into strips and grill them until they soften and become slightly translucent. Grilled banana squash is a great substitute for french fries (the color is similar), but you will lose your taste for potatoes soon and never want to go back.

EXERCISE
Do absolutely nothing.

Sunday

BREAKFAST
Have fresh fruit and a scrambled egg.

LUNCH

Make grilled salmon with broccoli and celery. Drizzle them with olive oil and balsamic vinegar and sprinkle fresh garlic and Asian red chilies on top. The omega-3 oils in the fish will reduce the inflammatory toxins that may be released from the fat cells you are eliminating from your body as you lose weight.

DINNER

After a weekend of good eating, Sunday is a perfect day to skip dinner. Most of you will probably anticipate this with some fear, and so you'll load up at lunch. This is OK, but you will get over it and eventually will randomize your meal-skipping so even you can't anticipate the next time you'll go hungry. If you feel dizziness or ravenously hungry, those are signs that your metabolism has been damaged by years of carbohydrate abuse. Be sure not to drive in this condition (one reason I start you on a Sunday evening). Dizziness may indicate dehydration (something you should not have because you drink to thirst and do not do long hours of training) so it likely means low glucose. To curb this feeling, eat a bit of dark chocolate or a piece of fruit. Back that up with an egg white (from your hard-boiled stash). Just remind yourself that your ancestors endured many episodes of hunger and that your metabolism is designed to handle brief fasts.

EXERCISE

Instead of eating dinner, take a walk. Or join a gym that's convenient to home or work and start weight training. Find a good instructor and begin to learn your way around. Activity is a signal to your metabolism to retain muscle even in the face of an energy shortage. Fasting and intense exercise both cause your body to release growth hormone, which makes fatty acids available to fuel your workout. The hunger from missing dinner will go away, and you will become a pure fat burner.

On Monday morning you will be getting compliments or stares from slightly envious friends in the office. You will look and feel younger and stronger. You will have more energy because your brain will be well fed and your mitochondria—those little energy furnaces in all your cells—will begin to regenerate as you relieve the glucose assault to which they have been subjected.

At this point, the sabotage may begin. Your friends will have noticed that you are eating in what they consider to be a strange way. It always happens. Don't bother to explain your appearance or eating to them, since they will only argue with you to bring you back to eating in a way they feel comfortable with.

Every female I know who has followed the diet has experienced this phenomenon. When we were dating, my wife lost five dress sizes in a matter of a few months, and her co-workers started saying, "You're too skinny" and brought her baked goods and other sugary treats. I think they were trying to undermine her. It also happens to guys in the gym who aren't doing their cardio training anymore. Their buddies tell them they're crazy. But it's all nonsense.

You'll have noticed that I do not specify portion size in this eating plan. That's because nobody but you knows what your energy intake and expenditures are. So how could anyone possibly tell you how much you should eat? Once your metabolism is functioning properly again, your appetite will become a healthy guide to your energy intake. I have weighed 200 pounds for more than 50 years and I have never counted my caloric intake or my energy expenditures. Nor do I use anything other than my appetite to limit how much I eat.

The low-energy density of the New Evolution Diet and the filling nature of the food (it is nearly impossible to overeat), mixed with intermittent, brief fasts, are more than enough to manage your energy intake. As your body composition improves, your appetite will determine your eating appropriately.

Week 2

Monday

BREAKFAST

Slices of avocado, lean turkey breast, one-quarter of an apple, and grapes.

LUNCH

Shrimp or tuna (canned or fresh) mixed with olives, leeks, and big chunks of celery drizzled with olive oil and flavored vinegar.

DINNER

Grilled lean flank steak, lightly marinated in homemade barbecue sauce (cook tomatoes and fresh chili peppers until they form a thick sauce). If you feel as though you've been eating too much red meat, replace the steak with skinless chicken breast or pork chops. Steam or sauté broccoli or asparagus.

EXERCISE

Lift weights at the gym or at home. Or sprint in a field or cycle at a rapid pace on a stationary bike. If you use a bike, see how many watts you can generate in a gentle but maximum effort. Then make two attempts to exceed that number.

Tuesday

BREAKFAST

One whole egg and two egg whites scrambled with bits of Italian sausage, tomato, and mushrooms. Add a large slice of honeydew melon with a few dark red grapes.

LUNCH

Lean turkey breast along with a salad of tomatoes dressed in olive oil and a few small chunks of mozzarella cheese, for taste.

DINNER

Salmon steak grilled or blackened with red peppers and artichokes or spinach, topped with slices of avocado and hot chilies. Make coleslaw with raw red and white cabbage mixed with white vinegar, olive oil, and a few chili flakes. Make a big batch, mix it, and let chill before you eat it.

EXERCISE

Lie on your back in a field or your yard and look up at the sky. Just do nothing as you watch the clouds or stars. Reading or watching television is not "doing nothing." Our ancestors had plenty of time to do nothing. It quiets our brains and reduces stress hormone levels. Doing nothing is even better than meditation because you don't have to control and quiet your brain as you do when you meditate. You want to get outside yourself, not more deeply inside.

Wednesday

BREAKFAST

Leftover flank steak or salmon from Monday or Tuesday. Have a small bunch of red grapes.

LUNCH

Sauerkraut with two large, grilled frankfurters. I know that hot dogs are supposed to be toxic, but I eat them now and then. The large ones taste much better than the small ones; I keep the large, better tasting ones around for a quick snack. Find frankfurters that are low in salt and fat. Otherwise, eat your sauerkraut with grilled pork loin.

DINNER

When our store has lobster tail or fresh crab legs, we buy them. Serve them with a tomato salad made with thin red onion slices, basil, and olive oil.

EXERCISE

If you have children, buy a thick, soft rope that's 8 to 12 feet long. Take them to a field and play tug-of-war. When I do this with my grandchildren, every kid in the park comes over to help my grandchildren try to beat me. I end up with a good workout. And the kids love it.

Hug your wife and lift her carefully off the ground, or move something you have been meaning to relocate or get rid of. Pick up a small child and walk around the house. Climb stairs or play with your children or dogs.

Thursday

BREAKFAST

An omelet cooked with onion or leftover broccoli or asparagus. A few slices of bacon, well cooked and drained. Add a handful of red raspberries or any fresh fruit of the season.

LUNCH

A few fresh steamed shrimp with celery slices, a bit of tomato and red onion salad, and avocado drizzled lightly with olive oil and flavored vinegar.

DINNER

Grill a skewer with pork and beef, red onion, and red peppers. Steam two broccoli florets and toss a large salad with romaine lettuce, avocado, celery, and olives. Make your own Italian dressing with dried packaged spices (available in the supermarket) mixed with olive oil and balsamic vinegar.

EXERCISE

Take a medicine ball outside and toss it as high up as you can, as though you are shooting a free throw. Move out of the way as it falls. Then throw it as far forward as you can and sprint after it. Then throw it sideways, sprint to it, and throw it back over your head. (Be careful with this maneuver: Don't use your lower back as a hinge; instead, stand straight, bend at the hips, and use your legs.)

Friday

BREAKFAST

Two thin pork chops grilled in a pan with fresh rosemary. A few slices of watermelon or cantaloupe are refreshing with this.

LUNCH

Fresh or canned tuna over lettuce and tomatoes, sprinkled with sliced spring onions and Italian dressing. Or use your homemade, fresh cole-slaw as a bed under the fish.

DINNER

Salmon steak grilled in a pan with celery, olives, broccoli, and slices of leek, mushrooms, and red chilies. Make a sauce with lemon and a little melted butter. Butter is OK now and then; it contains a wide range of vitamins and only a few of the potentially damaging milk proteins and lactose (milk sugar).

EXERCISE

Practice the abdominal brace and take a walk, preferably in the cool air so you get just a hint of a chill. Cold *is* exercise. Brown fat (adipose) tissues are furious fat burners when stimulated by cool temperatures. Exercise increases the expression of a protein, UCP, found in brown fat and muscle that makes you burn fat more efficiently.

Saturday

BREAKFAST
Dinner leftovers with cantaloupe slices and a few red grapes.

LUNCH
Have a handful of unsalted mixed nuts with a small chunk of Jarlsberg, a low-fat cheese made with skim milk and not much salt.

DINNER
Have a huge plate of steamed mussels with artichoke hearts sautéed in olive oil with a big salad of mixed greens, sliced bok choy, olives, and chunks of avocado.

EXERCISE
Do something to raise your insulin sensitivity before dinner: Take a brief walk or climb a few flights of stairs. You get hungry in anticipation of eating because your brain instructs your pancreas to release insulin, which lowers your blood sugar and triggers hunger. So even thinking about food makes your body hungry. There's nothing to fear, of course, since dinner is coming soon, even though your brain chemistry may tell you to eat right *now*. Knowing how your brain affects your hormones gives you some freedom to act as you wish, rather than being driven by a frightened brain. You probably won't starve to death, but your brain doesn't know that, and so it acts on its most primitive fear.

Sunday

BREAKFAST
A bacon and egg white omelet with fruit.

LUNCH
A small shrimp cocktail with avocado and celery drizzled with olive oil and flavored vinegar.

DINNER
A large steak with sautéed spinach and half a microwaved yam. I know I've said to steer clear of tubers, but a small yam once in a while is fine. Add on a romaine salad topped with thin slices of white onion, almonds, Italian dressing, and a few anchovies.

EXERCISE
Before dinner, hike in the wildest park you can find.

Week 3

Monday

BREAKFAST
Leftover steak with grapes or blueberries.

LUNCH
Homemade egg salad made with just a touch of mayonnaise. On the side, romaine with red onion slices and black and green olives with your homemade Italian dressing. Have a few cantaloupe slices.

DINNER
Barbecued spareribs or pork loin with a steamed fresh artichoke.

EXERCISE
Lift weights at the gym or at home. I like to tie a rope to my Range Rover and try pulling it, as though I am hauling a carcass back from a

hunt. I pull it partway up the slope of my driveway a few times almost every week. Now and then my wife will pull it too, just a few feet.

Tuesday

BREAKFAST
Two hard-boiled eggs, slices of avocado and cantaloupe, and a few red grapes.

LUNCH
A light salad with celery, red cabbage, red onion, and avocado, along with a few bits of leftover meat or fish.

DINNER
Let's eat out. Maybe a grilled steak covered with steamed crab and asparagus, plus a small side salad with no croutons; always try to avoid croutons, which are oxidized stale bread and oils.

EXERCISE
Sprint for 10 seconds on a stationary bike, then pedal smoothly for 20 to 30 seconds, and then sprint a bit harder for another 10 seconds. Do this four to six times, racing a bit harder each time, until you are maxing out by the last sprint. I assume you have your doctor's clearance to exercise. Heart patients are rehabilitated with high-intensity (but brief) training. It is far safer, and more effective, than jogging.

Wednesday

BREAKFAST
A bit of the leftover barbecued spareribs with fresh cantaloupe slices and a few red grapes for color.

LUNCH
Fresh or packaged smoked salmon over fresh spinach, green olives, romaine lettuce, celery, and tomato with pine nuts sprinkled on top.

DINNER
Fresh steamed mussels in a red marinara sauce with a steamed artichoke and an olive oil and balsamic vinegar dip with hot chili pepper.

EXERCISE
Your choice: Either lift weights for 15 minutes or just do nothing for half an hour, lying on your back, gazing at the ceiling or sky.

Thursday

BREAKFAST
Skip breakfast.

LUNCH
Heart of romaine with freshly cooked bacon, anchovies, olives, tomato, and red chili flakes topped with Italian dressing.

DINNER
A large swordfish steak grilled in olive oil and garlic with broccoli, red cabbage, celery, fresh white mushrooms, and spring onion. A small mixed green salad with avocado and thin slices of raw carrot.

EXERCISE
Play basketball before dinner or walk up several flights of stairs.

Friday

BREAKFAST
Bacon leftovers from yesterday's lunch with some cantaloupe, avocado, and a few red grapes.

LUNCH
Fresh chicken breast on sliced tomatoes and onions with homemade Italian dressing.

DINNER
Go out to a restaurant you like and pick something fresh, healthy, and delicious.

EXERCISE
Do nothing at all.

Saturday

BREAKFAST
Watermelon, red grapes, and a 100% beef frankfurter sliced and served with two scrambled eggs.

LUNCH
Turkey breast over fresh spinach, sprinkled with tomato slices, red onions, leeks, and hot green chilies with a few slices of fresh strawberries for color.

DINNER
New York strip steak with a great vegetable, like leeks grilled with banana squash.

EXERCISE

Stand up during the commercials when you watch TV. Begin to adopt that as a habit. Sitting is not not-exercising. Prolonged sitting is damaging because it interrupts fat metabolism.

Sunday

BREAKFAST

Chunks of pear and watermelon with sliced, lean pepper-coated turkey breast (this is always in our refrigerator for a quick meal or snack, though we seldom snack).

LUNCH

Frozen cooked shrimp, thawed but cold, with tomatoes, red onions, leeks, a bit of kale, and two stalks of celery with dark olives. Dressing to taste.

DINNER

A large grilled pork loin and a large mixed green salad made up of raw red cabbage slices, tomato, and big chunks of very fresh celery.

EXERCISE

Get outside when it's sunny and wear shorts and a T-shirt. Sunshine is a vitamin.

Week 4

Monday

BREAKFAST

Leftover pork loin with cantaloupe. I may eat as much as 10 ounces of lean pork loin at breakfast.

LUNCH

A homemade fish or chicken taco topped with romaine lettuce, slices of fresh red and white cabbage, and slices of jalapeño, all on a large tortilla toasted in a pan. Eat as little of the tortilla as possible, but enjoy what you eat of it.

DINNER

One of my most-often repeated meals: spareribs on the grill with artichokes and a romaine salad.

EXERCISE

Take up a sport long neglected, or start one you've always wanted to try—preferably one that makes you move, like basketball or tennis.

Tuesday

BREAKFAST

Eggs with bacon, a few grapes, and half a pear.

LUNCH

Chunks of leftover grilled pork loin over mixed salad greens with leek and celery slices and olives. Use olive oil and a little balsamic vinegar as a dressing and sprinkle the salad with dried chili pieces.

DINNER

Lightly grilled cod over a bed of Bibb lettuce with shrimp and steamed broccoli.

EXERCISE

Go into the gym you joined earlier and find a good instructor to show you around. In the next chapter, I will show you how to do it my way. Just know for now that it is the fountain of youth for men and women.

Wednesday

BREAKFAST
Three small, thin pork chops sautéed in olive oil with thin slices of white onion and chunks of honeydew and apple.

LUNCH
One can of smoked oysters over lettuce with snow peas and sliced green olives with jalapeño.

DINNER
Large cooked, packaged shrimp with avocado slices over a bed of romaine lettuce and kale. We serve it with olive oil and balsamic vinegar for dressing and shrimp sauce on the side.

EXERCISE.
Toss a football with a child or friend.

Thursday

BREAKFAST
Two hard-boiled eggs, two slices of well-cooked, drained bacon, and a few fresh strawberries and grapes.

LUNCH
Grilled chicken breast with a salad of romaine lettuce, artichoke hearts, and red cabbage with bits of bacon and Italian dressing.

DINNER
Egg drop soup made with chicken broth into which you put some spinach, tomato, and bits of crabmeat. Alongside that, stir-fry broccoli and sliced beef with hot chilies and a dash of low-sodium teriyaki sauce.

EXERCISE

Second session of weight training. Focus on learning the equipment and the basic exercises from your instructor. Forget what they tell you about how to eat. Don't "do your cardio," as they may suggest.

Friday

BREAKFAST

Almonds with avocado and three hard-boiled eggs. Eat just one or two of the yolks.

LUNCH

Sliced beef in a romaine salad sprinkled with a little shredded provolone cheese, tomato, and red onion slices. We buy precooked, packaged beef and use it often in salads for lunch or with fruit for breakfast. Packaged pulled pork is very useful and quick; just leave off some of the sauce.

DINNER

Halibut sautéed and placed hot over fresh spinach (this will wilt the spinach). Sautéed asparagus with a large romaine salad with hearts of palm and olives.

EXERCISE

Do nothing.

Saturday

BREAKFAST

A ham steak lightly grilled with a few slices of watermelon, a piece of pear, and a few red grapes.

LUNCH

Pepper-coated smoked turkey breast with avocado.

DINNER

When we shop at the grocery store, we often buy a precooked whole rotisserie chicken and take it home to serve with any fresh vegetable that looks good that day in the store.

EXERCISE

Take an easy walk in the morning when it is chilly (don't bundle up).

Sunday

BREAKFAST

Leftover chicken with avocado slices.

LUNCH

Shrimp over lettuce, with a salad of hard-boiled egg slices, celery, green olives, and artichoke hearts.

DINNER.

Skip dinner.

EXERCISE

Walk easily for 20 minutes instead of eating.

The Worst Foods You Can Eat

I have strong views on how to eat because it is crucial to health. But I try not to demonize particular foods, even ones that are very bad for us. I tend to be a libertarian in these matters; you should know the facts, then make your own choices. However, I am deeply concerned with how people feed their children. Many of my Web site members feed their children the New Evolution Diet with wonderfully positive results. When our grandchildren come to visit, my wife and I give them the same food we eat, and they love it.

But not everyone feeds children this way. In fact, there is one dish in particular—beloved by juvenile palettes and ubiquitous on children's menus—that is, in my view, the absolute worst food a human being can eat.

A few years ago, my wife and I were having an early supper at one of her favorite restaurants, a place called The Cheesecake Factory. (It is a testament to the ease with which one can follow our diet that you can find plenty to eat at a place with such a name.) We shared the artichoke appetizer, which was steamed and then grilled with a balsamic and olive oil dip, and we split a Caesar salad, no croutons. We each also had the combination steak Diane and crusted salmon entrée with asparagus on the side. No bread.

I looked over to my right and saw a family of seven being served a big mound of brown food. That was the only color on the table—a bad sign. Color is a reliable guide to nutritious, well-balanced meals. The more colors on the table, and the brighter they are, the better the eating.

This family included multiple generations, from grandparents to small children. Every plate was nearly covered by a large mound of french fries. Their monochromatic meal included the dark brown of a hamburger here and there and the blackish brown of the Cokes they were drinking.

The sight of it ruined my dinner.

I am used to seeing children being fed french fries by their parents. It is a cheap dish. Kids love them, and they're always on the children's menu no matter where you go. Nearly every kiddie meal at a fast-food restaurant features french fries and a toy, giving potatoes yet another happy association in the mind of a child. Children today have a Pavlovian response to french fries; they signify dining out amid familial love and toys and pleasant experiences.

They also mean big trouble. A french fry is little more than a carbohydrate vessel for fat.[1] A combined carb-fat load would have been an extremely rare event in the nutritional history of our species. In ancestral times of 100,000 years ago, fat would have accompanied protein—not a simple carb. Our metabolic networks must be stressed by this combination. The carbs prompt our bodies to release insulin, which shuts down fat burning. The resulting high-fat load and high blood sugar becomes a heavy sludge in the bloodstream, bruising the lining of our blood vessels.

The release of insulin also opens this lining to the intrusion of fats. These fats are then oxidized, driven by the inflammatory response to high blood glucose. Oxidizing fat on a stream of glucose-mediated free radicals inflames the vasculature, promoting cardiovascular disease.

I really hate it when I see a kid eating french fries. I love my grandchildren too much to buy them fries. I hope they learn to associate vegetables, good health, and good food with their PaPa. When I take them out, I let them order from the adult menu. It is more expensive, but it is worth it to teach them about good food.

Fries aren't the only food to steer clear of. Here is my list of the Worst Foods You (and Your Children) Can Eat. Most of these foods alter your metabolism unfavorably or promote a stress response in your body.

10. **Pizza.** The only virtues of this mixture of fats and carbohydrates are the fresh tomatoes and spices some restaurants use.

9. **Wheat bread.** Not only is wheat bread high in gluten; it is also usually sweetened, because the acids in the wheat make the bread bitter.

8. **Soy sauce and other soy products.** As I've mentioned, highly processed soy products can raise estrogen levels in men and women, causing damaging health effects. Highly processed soy products also pack a big hit of sodium.

7. **Refried beans.** This Mexican-restaurant favorite is full of lectins and toxins (they are partially detoxified by cooking, but never completely) as well as carbohydrates and fats, the worst combination of nutrients.

6. **Rice.** Unlike brown rice or wild rice, which contain fiber and essential B complex vitamins, refined white rice offers little nutritional value. The color white should generally be avoided in foods; think white refined flour, white bread, and sugar. Eating white is like putting up the surrender flag and signalling you give up on protecting your metabolism.

5. **Casseroles.** Who knows what's in these starchy, greasy dishes? It's usually a mixture of carbs, fats, and dairy with no fresh vegetables or other healthy ingredients. Avoid this mystery food.

4. **Processed white flour.** Nearly all baked goods contain this ingredient, to which hydrogenated oils are added to hold the thing together, create texture, and ensure shelf life. The result is a mixture of unnatural trans fats with altered proteins that humans never consumed until a few decades ago.

3. **Energy bars and drinks, trail mix, soft drinks, and sports drinks.** These are things that endurance athletes typically consume in abundance. So do our children and those who would emulate athletes. Most of these products, particularly soft drinks and sports drinks, contain a mixture of sodium and sugar. The sugar hides the taste of the salt, and the salt makes you thirsty. So you drink some more as you dehydrate, and the acids in the drinks, which provide flavor, are acidic enough to erode your teeth (water has a pH of 7.0, sodas have an average pH of 2.38). To buffer the acid, the body takes calcium from your bones.

2. **Foods and drinks containing artificial sweeteners.** Diet sodas and other "diet" foods and drinks induce hunger because both the brain and the stomach respond to the extreme sweetness of artificial sweeteners by releasing insulin, which makes blood sugar drop and increases hunger.

1. **High-fructose corn syrup and cereal.** In a tie, these are the worst things you can eat (next to french fries). High-fructose corn syrup (HCFS) promotes an altered metabolic cycle that depletes adenosine triphosphate (ATP), the universal fuel in the body. So, even though HCFS contains energy, it leaves you with less energy because of this odd metabolic quirk. As a result, you get hungry and eat more. In addition, this liquid corn sugar is metabolized primarily in the liver, leaving droplets of fat with each hit. What do you call something that has no utilizable energy and is metabolized primarily in the liver? A toxin, according to many scientists.

Anything found in the cereal section of the supermarket— where our children get a large portion of their energy consumption—is also a food to avoid. Aside from chips, processed, sweetened cereals contain less nutrition per calorie than just about any other food you can find. Whole-grain cereals generally provide twice the amount of nutrients than refined cereal products, but at twice the price.

Many parents view cereals as a healthy snack food for their young children, but in fact at least one study has indicated that infants who consume fortified cereals (cereals that contain added vitamins) are at some risk of excess nutrient intake. This is important because some nutrients—such as vitamin A, zinc, folate—appear to have the potential for toxic levels of intake. It's also been shown that noninfant cereals—in other words, "adult" cereals—are among the grain products most commonly consumed by toddlers over the age of 12 months. And while most toddlers are eating nonpresweetened cereals (defined as cereals with less than 21.2 grams of sugar per 100-gram serving), between 18 and 26 percent of toddlers age 12 months or older are eating presweetened cereals.[2]

So from a very early age, we're exposing our children to an array of substances our Paleolithic ancestors would not have even recognized, let alone consumed. If we want our children to live long, healthy lives, it's time to start feeding them real foods.

Some cereals are "fortified," meaning vitamins are added. When you see that word, you know that the product itself contains nothing of value. Mix sugary, low-nutrient cereal with milk and you have a combination of assaults on the body that humans never faced through eons of evolution.

CHAPTER 6

How to Exercise

Today is a gym day for me. I'd like you to come along.

I visit the gym anywhere between one and four times a week, depending on how I feel. When I work out hard, I may take 2 or 3 days off to recover.

My gym routine also varies because I want to keep my workouts a little random and unplanned. Too much regimentation in exercise is a bad thing, regardless of what you've been led to believe.[1]

I spend as little time as possible working out, usually no more than half an hour or so. That's all anybody needs. I also keep my gym visits to a minimum to avoid boredom. There are nicer places to be and finer things to do with your life than hang around gyms. It's possible to exercise too much.[2]

Here's another good reason to keep your workouts short: The physical stress causes the release of adrenaline, noradrenalin, glucocorticoids, along with inflammatory cytokines, such as tumor necrosis factor alpha, IL-1, and IL-6. These serve to maintain blood glucose and fatty acids to be used as energy and to maintain blood pressure and optimize the delivery of energy (ATP) to muscle at the expense of other tissues. Short-term stress, of the fight-or-flight kind we experience in short, intense bouts of exercise, activates the mitochondria (the energy furnaces in each cell) and increases their output and number. Prolonged stress causes dysfunction and abnormalities in the mitochondria that may lead to the death of the cell they reside in. But if the intense exertion goes on for long, the body will release another stress hormone, cortisol, which we don't want, at least not now. Excessive cortisol secretion is associated with high blood pressure, depression, immune suppression, osteoporosis, and metabolic syndrome. (It will be released, moderately, later if we keep the exercise brief. This is unavoidable, and is associated with turning down the stress response and the release of IL-6, which helps to reduce muscle inflammation acutely, but not chronically.) This all makes perfect evolutionary sense, since stresses 40,000 years ago tended to be of the short-term, fight-or-flight variety, where the acute stress response was essential to our survival.

I go to the gym in the morning, not long after I wake up, for the simple reason that a workout is more effective if done on an empty stomach. You burn more energy this way. Sometimes I have a cup of coffee first, but nothing more; the caffeine starts the adrenaline flowing, increases blood flow to the muscle, and mobilizes glucose for burning.

That, too, runs counter to what you may have been taught. The idea that you should eat first—the "experts" usually counsel a big helping of carbs, supposedly to fuel your muscles—is actually counterproductive if burning fat is among your goals. Later I'll explain why it is better not only to exercise hungry but also to put off eating afterward for up to an hour.

The main goal here is to reach for intensity. I don't want this to sound scary, but each workout needs to take you to an extreme. Your body should be required to do something it has never done before. I've seen people who turn their gym workout into a routine as predictable as any other, like a task they can do on autopilot. They don't realize they need to push themselves, so they settle for a mildly taxing session that pretty much replicates all the workouts they've done before.[3]

This defeats the entire purpose of exercise. You should be looking for an experience that will change you, inside and out. Each workout is supposed to leave its mark on you, alter you—to make you a better specimen of human being than you were when you walked in the door. And that's only possible if your exertions reach the point of intensity.

That doesn't mean you need to devote a great deal of time to exercising, however. Professor James Timmons, of Heriot-Watt University in Edinburgh, Scotland, tested the effect of what he termed "high-intensity interval training" on the metabolisms of sedentary male volunteers. His findings include evidence that "doing a few intense muscle exercises, each lasting only about 30 seconds, dramatically improves your metabolism in just two weeks." Precisely my point.[4]

Here's what one of my blog readers had to report on the subject: "I am a medical doctor and have exercised all my life, tolerating quite horrible muscle soreness and poor recovery. I was immediately attracted by the logic of the diet but took longer to fully appreciate the exercise recommendations. At 38 I am stronger, faster, leaner and more alert than I've ever been. Muscle stiffness is virtually a thing of the past, as are hunger and cravings. My 'formal' exercise sessions (as opposed to play) total 50 minutes a week. I couldn't recommend this more."

The first thing I do at the gym is head for a stationary bike. You need to warm up your heart, as well as your core temperature, before the real work begins. When you increase your core temperature, the pituitary gland responds by releasing growth hormone. That event is vital to a successful workout: The hormone mobilizes fat to burn for the rest of your session, and even beyond.

Unlike most people at the gym, however, I don't stay on the bike for long—just 6 minutes total, which is enough time to break a sweat and get a good burn going, if you ride as I do. First, I pedal with low resistance at a fast sprint. After 1 minute of that, I turn the resistance up to the maximum possible and ride just as hard as I can for the next 60 seconds. I repeat that pattern twice more—a minute of sprinting at low resistance, followed by one that feels as though I am riding through peanut butter. During that sixth minute, I do my best to max out the meter that measures watts of energy expended. Then I'm done.

Professor Leila Barraj's research actually shows that doing just 7 minutes *a week* on a stationary bike, riding intensely as I do, can make significant improvements in your ability to metabolize glucose. Other studies show that intermittent, intense sprinting can double endurance capacity in 2 weeks. It's the intensity that counts, not the duration. Other research shows that intensity is the key to having a body that is lean.

Anyway, enough warm-up. Time to move along.

The very idea of exercise is alien and unnatural to every life-form, us included. No wonder we have such a hard time with it. Either we do too little, or we do it badly—even to the point of harming ourselves with an activity intended to be beneficial.

Perhaps that's because it *is* such an artificial pursuit. I don't mean to say that exertion is unnatural. It is what we are built to do. Our genes are adapted to an existence of hard physical work, and when we fulfill that potential properly, they reward us by expressing themselves in a healthy way.

But remember that from an evolutionary perspective, humans are lazy overeaters. We survived as a species only by exerting ourselves as little as possible (and thereby conserving energy, back when it was scarce). For most of the time we've existed, our environment has been challenging enough to keep us strenuously active. Thanks to civilization, the world has changed a great deal since our genes stopped evolving. But even all the laborsaving technology we've invented is a mixed blessing: By solving one set of problems, it has created another. We ignore our genetic legacy when we label the obese as lazy and unwilling to limit their food intake.[5]

So these are the questions facing us today: How do we motivate an essentially lazy genotype to exert itself? And what form should our exertions take?

As always, we can look back and deduce what kinds of activity our prehistoric forebears practiced. Then we can attempt to replicate it here and now.

There is no doubt that the hunter-gatherers were strong—stronger than we are. Their remains are very revealing. Cro-Magnon and Neanderthal left extremely robust skeletons, with huge attachment points for the muscles, which implies exceptional strength. The bones are dense and highly mineralized. The poor Neanderthal has a skeleton that resembles that of a rodeo cowboy, full of injuries and evidence of arthritis from repetitive injury stress, including breaks that healed. Neanderthal must have lived up close with the animals they hunted, because they only had heavy spears, which were suitable for thrusting rather than throwing. Cro-Magnon, on the other hand, left behind a taller, less robust skeleton that is relatively free of injuries. It is known that they had spears they could throw, and even implements that would propel the spear farther. And, at some point, they used bows and arrows.

We can also look to contemporary hunter-gatherer tribes for evidence of ancient activity patterns. Until the introduction of snowmobiles and rifles, the Native Alaskan Inuit tribes hunted for seals and whales in traditional ways. First came many hours of quiet exploration and searching, followed by intense moments of the kill. Even butchering and hauling the prey back to camp required brute strength and aerobic capacity.

There are compelling stories of the Native American's physical exertions as well. Their diet was largely composed of buffalo meat, and they ate, on average, 4 pounds of it a day. They hunted buffalo in two ways: They ran them off cliffs, and they rode horses alongside them and speared them. The Spanish explorer Vasco da Gama wrote of meeting a Native American who was allegedly 7 feet tall and powerfully muscled and could run alongside buffalo himself to spear them. He may have been exaggerating, but keep in mind that the Spaniard had come from a continent populated mainly by scrawny, malnourished farmworkers. The physical strength and beauty of Native Americans made an impression on their European colonizers, who shipped many "specimens" back to Europe for display.

An anthropologist who visited the Aché of Paraguay—a tribe of hunters who move through the forest continuously, hunting peccary—was shocked to discover that more than half the adult males in the group could outrun him, including men he estimated to be in their fifties. The anthropologist in question was a sub-11-second sprinter in college.[6] The Aché go quietly through the forest at a brisk walking or jogging pace and then sprint when their prey is close at hand. The men consume roughly 5,000 calories daily—a huge amount. They need all that energy to keep going. We require less than half that to get through our sedentary days.

Physically and genetically, we are built to run fast and climb trees easily. But few of us over the age of 11 do so. Which is why we're now at the gym.

After the bike I head for the leg machines. Because the hamstring muscles—the biceps femoris—are so large, working them first keeps my body temperature up. And the lactate they release tells the pituitary to keep pumping out growth hormone.

First up are leg curls. Most gyms have weight machines for this exercise, done either seated or lying facedown. In each case, you start with straight legs and then bend the knees to bring your feet closer to the back of your thighs.

Most people choose a suitably challenging weight and then do two or three sets of 8 to 10 repetitions, with a minute's break between sets. Instead, I build my sets in a hierarchy, like this: First, 15 repetitions using a relatively light weight, which I move slowly. That starts the burn, which is the sign I'm looking for. Then, I get up, add more weight—maybe a third of what was on there—and without taking a break, do 8 reps, a little more quickly than the first round. Finally, I add still more weight, up around my maximum, and do 4 reps, quickly. And that's that.

There's a good reason for this hierarchy of repetitions and weight levels. It matches the sequence in which your three main types of muscle fibers go to work. The slow-twitch fibers go first—they exhaust themselves on the first set, with light weights and a high number of reps. The slow-twitch fibers primarily burn fat. On the second set, they recruit the intermediate-twitch muscles for assistance—and they, too, are used up. Those muscles burn both glycogen and fat. You need to push through slow- and intermediate-twitch fibers first in order to summon the grade-A stuff: the fast-twitch fibers. Intense exercise is challenging and productive (exceeding 10 METS is considered to be "very hard" exercise—equivalent to a run, but short bursts of sprinting can exceed 25 METS, something I do often). They go to work on the final, heaviest set. They are the ones you want to mobilize, since they burn glycogen now and, later during recovery, they burn fat—in fact, they burn from three (the FTa fibers) to four (the FTx fibers) times as much energy as the slow-twitch fibers. They are also the most valuable muscle fibers when it comes to strength and body composition. Essentially, to be strong means to have plenty of fast-twitch muscle fiber.

The conventional wisdom requires you to wait a minute or even more between sets—"recovery time," as it is called. This, too, is wrongheaded, in my opinion. There's no advantage in letting muscle recover too much; the point here is to work it hard. You want to burn off the blood sugar, or glycogen, contained in your muscles as quickly as you can. And you need intense work to do that.

Once the glycogen is gone, the lactic acid floods in. That seems to be what causes the familiar "burn." That painful sensation tells me that my body is using glycogen and the lactic acid that has been released by the exercise. Whatever the source of the burn (which is in dispute) you want to hit the lactate threshold so you learn to use lactate as a fuel and exhaust or deplete the glycogen stored in the muscle and use fat as the fuel for recovery. However, I do *not* perform an exercise "to failure," meaning the point at which I literally am unable to do another repetition. For a number of reasons, pushing a muscle to where it can do no more is a bad idea.

For one thing, doing that probably means you are struggling

through the last reps, breaking proper form, gritting your teeth, and potentially injuring a tendon or a joint as you heroically try to reach the point of total muscle exhaustion. It's unnecessary, and all that grunting is ugly on the ears.

Another reason I don't like the idea of working a muscle to failure is that you are at the gym to seek success, and the brain records every failure as exactly that: You failed. It's a bad habit, especially in pursuit of health.

After working the hamstrings, I go directly to the seated leg extension machine to balance out the movement I've just done. On this seated exercise, start with the knees bent and straighten them against resistance, working the front of the thigh. Again, I do this in the 15-8-4 rep sequence, adding weight and increasing speed with each set.

The final stop for the lower body workout: the leg press. There are several kinds; the seated one is best because it puts less stress on your back. Using it is also superior, for the same reason, to doing squats with a heavy barbell resting on your shoulders. But the action is essentially the same: pushing away a heavy load with both feet. This is a good measure of strength—men in good shape can move at least double their body weight in this exercise; women, a little less.

I will often do a variation on this by using both legs to push the weight out but just one to lower it. This is called a "negative" because most of the exertion is in the lowering, not the lifting. In every exercise, you can usually move about 40 percent more in the negative part of the movement than in the "positive," or lifting, phase, where you work against gravity. Lowering presents its own challenge because you're not fighting against gravity; you're just trying to slow it down.

A negative, in any exercise, is a great muscle builder. It actually tears the fibers, which isn't a bad thing—they then grow back larger and stronger than before. It's also called an eccentric movement. It is extremely taxing and should be done with care. Now we're through with the leg exercises. It's time to move along to the upper body workout.

A friend of mine, a retired Marine, had a heart attack during a long bicycle ride that was part of his training for an upcoming triathlon. I wrote about him on my blog:

> I think our Marines are about as tough and brave as anyone can be. A friend of mine is a retired Marine. When I first saw him about 2 years ago, he was tan and lean and had a shaved head. He looked terrific.
>
> When he came by my house last week I wondered what had happened to him. He was pale, kind of softish, with too much tissue hanging out everywhere, and limping. I asked him why. He said he'd pulled or tore a hamstring while running a 10-K. This is his third tear in 2 years.
>
> I knew he had been doing triathlons for the past 2 years, but I hadn't seen him up close for some time. I was sad and surprised to see how he looked.
>
> His tan is gone because he trains indoors, riding the stationary bike, logging miles on the treadmill, and swimming laps in the indoor pool. The hamstring tears have been nagging because he won't stop training or doing events. So he has a more or less constant limp.
>
> Why did he gain weight when he was exercising so much? Because he eats the kind of junk runners have been taught to rely on. He does all the carbo-load meals preceding each event. (Does anybody still believe loading works? Apparently, but the belief is bogus. Only a depleted muscle from over-training requires anything like a load. And the CHO [carbohydrate] load ramps up insulin and blood sugar, and interferes with growth hormone.) He eats every kind of CHO you can lay your hands on; potato chips are consumed in large quantities. (Does he know about trans fatty acids?) He may permanently damage his hypothalamus-pituitary-adrenal axis.

If I may blow my own horn for a second: Back when I first began researching these topics, "experts" still swore by the practice of carb loading before a workout or athletic event. When I warned against it, I was a lone voice in the wilderness. Today, smart runners and other athletes have by and large realized that it was a very bad idea and no longer consume mass quantities of cheap carbs before physical exertion.

We are made more for walking and sprinting than for jogging. The fact is, few hunters ever literally ran down prey over the marathon distance of 26.2 miles. American Indians could bring down a horse in a matter of a few days, but that was done primarily by spooking the animal and then trailing it at a distance. Our ancestors sometimes needed to sprint at the decisive moment, when closing in for the kill, although human ingenuity commonly worked better, as when hunters would drive their prey into traps or dead ends from which they could not escape. They definitely needed to sprint when they themselves were the prey. Beyond that, however, hunters lived by the sensible maxim that led our ancestors to exert no more effort than was absolutely necessary.

As in all exercise, intermittency and variety are the goals in aerobic workouts. You want to stop and start, go in an instant from walking to running at top speed for 40 or 50 yards, then amble along until the urge to sprint overtakes you again. When you do this, you exercise all the different types of muscle fiber, whereas joggers work mainly the slow- and intermediate-twitch kinds. Jogging also wastes time because you need to do it for long periods to see any benefit. Mixing up sprints with walks is safer for your heart, too. And there's less stress on your knees, ankles, hips, feet, and back.

You get a good cardio workout just by lifting weights, as I suggest, without a break between sets or stations. When you do it vigorously and with a sense of purpose, your heart will be pumping and your lungs will be working. If you still feel the need for more aerobic exercise, find a game or sport to play. Tennis, racquetball, and basketball are intense, stop-and-start activities, meaning they burn all three kinds of muscle fiber. And they have the added advantage of being fun.

Lately I've been playing a lot of tennis, maybe four times a week, which is all the running I need. When I do my sprints, I will go once a week to a nearby field and race 40 yards, then stop, and repeat this a few times. If I lived near the beach I'd go a couple of times a week and do my sprints on the dry, loose sand, not the wet, packed part. Then I'd take a leisurely stroll for 45 minutes or so. Sprinting first releases growth hormone, and so the body goes on burning fat as you walk afterward.

Here's another great aerobic workout: Simply jump as high as you can and land in a squat with your thighs parallel to the ground. Do a dozen of these in rapid succession and see how you feel.

I always take a 20-minute walk after dinner, no matter where I am, not to burn energy but for the pleasure of it. When I travel, I walk constantly, climb stairs when possible, and take my Rollerblades when I can. It's my way of exercising away from home.

If you enjoy it, basketball is a great game from the aerobic perspective, with constant moving, sprinting, stopping on a dime, jumping, and diving. Look at the physiques of professional athletes—no athlete's physique is as powerful as a basketball player's. Basketball players test as the leanest of all pros, with around 8 percent body fat. Only football receivers, defensive backs, and running backs come close. They, too, move in unpredictable, varied ways—jogging one second, running full-tilt the next, cutting, swerving, and stopping.

If you need more proof, go to a track meet, then tell me: Would you rather look like the milers or the sprinters? The distance runners are stringy, emaciated, haunted. The sprinters look like classical Greek statuary. Keep in mind that the first person to run a marathon, Pheidippides, collapsed and died at the end of his run. Marathon running actually suppresses the immune system. As I was writing this book, I read that three runners died during the Detroit Free Press marathon—one of them a 26-year-old man, another just 36, both in good health.

Finally, the fact that long bouts of intense aerobic exercise (such as marathons and triathlons) causes harmful oxidation should also be taken as a sign that, from an evolutionary perspective, our bodies are not well adapted to jogging. The mortality curve is J-shaped: It declines with exercise, hits a bottom, and then rises. The overexercised fare no better than the underexercised.

Walking and sprinting are the safest and most beneficial forms of aerobic exercise. Perhaps not coincidentally, they are also the most enjoyable. A sprint is exhilarating, childlike fun. It brings a taste of animalistic wildness and abandon to your workouts. And I shouldn't have to explain the pleasures of a nice, brisk walk outdoors.

My upper body training routine also starts with the biggest muscles, to keep the growth hormone flowing and the heart pumping. So let's begin with the back. There are many ways to work those muscles, but I'm going to start with a seated cable row, in a hierarchical 15-8-4 set. To balance that, I move next to a barbell row done in a steep, almost-standing position, rather than the usual bent-over pose, so I work the upper trapezius from a new angle to involve more neck and shoulder muscles. I don't do many of these, because I don't want to tax my cervical vertebrae. This is more of a finishing move than anything else, done to improve symmetry of the trunk.

A word here about that concept, symmetry. Having a well-balanced figure seems more a cosmetic concern than anything else, but it's not. You want to be strong all over, not just in some places. There are some exercises I do only for symmetry's sake. You will notice that I don't do an exercise that nearly everybody in the gym does routinely—bicep curls. For weight trainers, biceps are an obsession. They are "mirror muscles"—guys love working on their arms because arm muscles respond well to weight training and make an impressive show when you stare at yourself in the mirror.

But the fact is that many of the upper body exercises you'll do already work the biceps and triceps (the muscle on the back of the upper arms). And face it, in the course of your daily life, how much arm power do you really need? I do curls or work the triceps only when I look at myself and see an imbalance.

That symmetry should be everywhere—upper body to lower, front of limb to back. Males and females alike should be shaped like an X: broad at the shoulders and hips, narrow at the waist. From an evolutionary perspective, symmetry is a reliable indication of health. In children, developmental diseases result in body asymmetry.

For our purposes, symmetry means you're probably in good shape. It shows you've attained balance in movement and in muscle groups, so there is less chance of injury while working out.

After the barbell row exercise, I move on to the chest workout, specifically the upper part of the pectoral muscles, just under the collarbone, which is where you most need strength. I find that weight lifters devote too much effort to building a massive chest, especially with the bench press exercise. You don't need all that bulk. And it looks grotesque. Here I do an incline dumbbell press, sitting on a bench at a 45-degree angle and using dumbbells so each side of my body works individually.

Shoulders are important, but you've been working them all along in your upper body exercises, so there's just one upper body routine left to do: the lateral raise machine, which works the deltoids (the muscles at the very top of your arm). This is more of a finishing move than anything else, and I do it at one of those side lift machines. You don't want to punish the shoulder muscles too much, since they are prone to injury. Some days I do this as a negative exercise—I raise the weights with both arms but then lower them with just one.

I tend not to spend much time working abdominal muscles as such. Whether you feel it or not, we've been working them all along. That's because we do the abdominal brace in every exercise. This means we lightly contract the abdominal muscles and maintain proper curvature of the lower back at all times, to develop a kind of postural strength. Posture is a full-time event. And the most fatigue-resistant muscles you have—your abs and your spinal erectors—must be engaged in maintaining proper posture.

Also, we have been imposing asymmetric loadings on the trunk, which recruits the abdominal and trunk muscles along with the spinal muscles. We've done this by working one limb at a time in exercises such as the one-armed dumbbell row and the one-legged press.

But there is one abdominal exercise to do—and only one: an ab curl. I make this quite intense by contracting the abdominal muscles before beginning the exercise. The curl is done by lying flat on the floor or on an elevated bench, bending the knees, and placing the feet flat, just under the hips. Once in this position, raise the upper trunk from the pelvis to lift the shoulders. I imagine that I am pressing some object in front of me upward by holding my arms out and curling with the abdominal muscles. You can even increase the resistance by having someone resist the upward push in the arms and hands.

This exercise can be done from side to side as well as upward. By varying the direction, the intercostal muscles in the rib cage are strengthened. A "six pack" will appear if and when the fat underneath the skin in the abdominal region becomes thin enough.

Finally, whenever I walk, I focus on maintaining the abdominal brace posture. If you do this, your ab muscles will become very strong. But keep in mind that having large abdominal muscles is not necessarily desirable. They only look good when they are contracted.

That's my workout. We're through.

Some women I know won't even try weight training. They fear it will turn them thick and bulky. They wonder why they can't just stick with spinning, or yoga, or running.

But lifting weights is even more important for women than for men! Women need to preserve their skeletal (bone) mass if they want to avoid osteoporosis, and building muscle mass is the only way to do that. By now it's become commonplace—an elderly person falls and breaks a hip, rendering him or her permanently unable to walk. My mother broke both of her hips and was never the same. She underwent surgery to fix them, but hip operations involve a large loss of blood flow and seem to affect mental acuity.

Even better than surviving a fall, of course, is preventing one. And the best way to do that is to have sufficient muscle mass, especially the fast-twitch kind, to keep you upright. Women tend to have less of that than men because they have less muscle mass, which is why they need to do more to maintain it.

It's true for women (as for men) that putting your muscle under the acute stress of a weight-lifting session releases growth hormones, which does *not* make you look like a bodybuilder. But it does burn fat and increase your sensitivity to insulin, which stops your body from storing more fat in the future.

Women do not have sufficient testosterone to build serious muscle mass even if they wanted to. For that, they would need to inject testosterone or a related steroid. Working out with weights won't make you big—just lean and strong.

I've taken you along on one of my typical workouts at the gym. But as I've said repeatedly in this book, variety, randomness, and intermittency are necessary to maintaining good health. So there's really no such thing as a typical day at the gym for me. I've done my best to avoid dictating how you should structure your workouts. Giving you a routine to slavishly follow would defeat my purpose.

I actually have several different types of workouts I use at the gym. Here are two of my favorites:

- Eccentric workout: This uses negative movements, as described on page 96. It is an intense way to work out—as I said earlier, it tears and stretches the muscle fibers, thus making them grow back stronger and larger. This adaptation can be done for arms, delts, shoulders, chest, and legs. The principle is always the same: You can handle more weight in the lowering phase of an exercise than in the lifting phase. So you use both arms or legs to get the weight up, and then just one arm or leg to set it back down; focus on contracting the muscle against the stretch (stretch under contraction may be the most productive way to build muscle mass).

A muscle-building secret: Contracting against stretch has been my "secret" method for maintaining a large muscle mass for 50 years (I call it flex/stretch). Whenever I want to add a little muscle mass, I do two flex/stretch workouts a week of 15 minutes each for up to 4 weeks. You need to experiment a little to determine how much weight you can control in the downward phase. These exercises are best done on weight machines rather than with free weights, for safety's sake.

- Alactic workout: This workout does not cause lactic acid to be released into the muscle. I do just one repetition of an exercise, for five sets. I use a heavy weight, about as much as I am able to lift for that single rep. This is a hard workout, too—not for beginners. You have to be careful to avoid injury. But it builds a huge amount of strength in a short time.

Now that you're done with our workout, you might be tempted to reward yourself with a big meal. But that's a bad idea. Your body only begins to burn fat after the workout is over. This is why you shouldn't eat anything right before or after exercise. Eating shuts down the fat-burning phase. Replenishing the glycogen in the muscle with one of those sports drinks that contain so much sugar along with the protein also shuts down the growth hormone and leads to the release of insulin, all of which are counterproductive. A good workout elevates your insulin sensitivity for up to 10 hours, affording ample time for the entry of nutrients, including protein and glycogen, into the muscle.

Eating right after a workout also suppresses metabolic gene expression. Consuming a replenishment drink right after is an exerciser's "comfort food" that works with the stress hormones and insulin to move fat from subcutaneous locations into the abdominal region. If you go to the gym hungry and stay that way for an hour after you're through, you burn more fat and improve your hormonal state, therefore taking maximum advantage of all that hard work.

Exercise actually turns down the action of what is known as the obesity gene.[7] This gene's job is to "express" fat—that is, to ramp up metabolic pathways that lead to the production of fat cells. The New Evolution Diet turns down the expression of the obesity gene in four different ways. First, it reduces glucose and insulin. Second, it involves intermittent fasting, which turns down the obesity gene. Third, it involves brief, intense exercise, which reduces the gene's expression. Fourth, it increases expression of UCP and brown fat, big energy consumers. This approach has enabled me to maintain less than 8 percent body fat for more than 25 years.

That ratio of fat to muscle must be maintained in the correct zone—roughly 11 percent body fat for males, 17 percent for females—if you are going to have a shot at a vital old age. Losing fat and gaining muscle may actually increase your weight, since muscle is denser and heavier than fat. This is why measures such as weight or BMI, while important, are absolutely secondary to body composition.

The main thing to remember is that physical activity is not simply something you do to help you lose weight. It is a crucial component of how your body adapted to its environment, and it is absolutely necessary for good health. If you're not active, you are depriving your body of something as vital to it as food, water, and sunlight.

Also, there is the not-insignificant fact that exercise, if done properly, will maintain your body in the shape it was meant to take, meaning shoulders and hips larger than your waist (but not by much), whether you are male or female, and no protruding belly. Physical activity ensures your form will be as sleek and graceful as nature intended, skeleton and muscles evident (though not *too*), articulating your limbs and torso. We tell one another not to judge a book by its cover, but the truth is that a great deal can be determined about your health just by looking at you. Strong muscles unobstructed by excess fat, good posture, taut skin, skin color that is neither too pale nor too ruddy (a sure sign of inflammation), overall proper proportions, a general air of well-being—these are the signs we all recognize, instinctually, as being evidence of good health. You don't need an expert to tell you that.

The fact that you are alive is a remarkable thing. The odds against it are great. The genes you carry contain information from a continuous strand of surviving organisms that extends 2 billion years back in time. You are an improbable event, and your existence is testimony to the toughness and adaptability of the ancestral line whence you come. You are a survivor, well equipped to live and thrive. Recognize, however, that the world for which your genes encode a successful design does not exist today.

Your brain and body expect you to live a life of movement and action, of challenge and response, of variety and adaptation. Your brain still "sees" sensory inputs as though you are a hunter-gatherer and, at the instinctual level, directs your actions accordingly. Example: You freeze before a large audience because your ancestors, when exposed on open ground, increased their odds of surviving by freezing to escape detection. If you accept this, you will be more relaxed and less apt to punish yourself for things you do, or don't do (like get out and move around).

Variety and play are the essential human attributes. By keeping your workouts brief and exhilarating, you won't get bored. By adding lots of outdoor activity and play, you will enjoy the power and fitness you gain. If you start a new sport, or pick up one long neglected, you will see how the power you gain improves your play. The feedback between the training and your new power in the sport will be rewarding enough to stick with it.

I fail to see how anyone can train 5 or 6 days a week in the gym and for hours at a time. That is factory or agricultural work, not anything human beings were evolved to do. And the paradox is that you will gain less strength and fitness if you overtrain. You will join the thousands who quit exercising out of sheer boredom. Overtraining increases your stress level, interferes with your sleep, raises your level of stress hormones, and reduces your level of growth hormones and testosterone. It leads to less muscle gain, not more, along with loss of fitness and boredom. Boredom is one way your brain stops you from harming yourself.[8]

As for goals, don't set any. The ones you are likely to choose are not functional. You will say I want to lose x pounds, but you really want to lose fat, not lean body mass. You want to eat the New Evolution Diet and move like an athlete to express the evolutionarily "normal" physiology of our hunter-gatherer ancestors.

You can't control the outcome, only the process. Just accept that what you are doing is what your body and mind were made to do, and that this active and metabolically challenging lifestyle is how it is going to be from now on.

Boys to Girls

In recent years a mysterious trend has been reported: Testosterone levels in men are dropping.[1] Not coincidentally, during that same period, the incidence of obesity has reached epidemic proportions. It amazes me that so few experts have made a connection between the poor diet of young men and the declining levels of the essential male hormone.

You'd think the guys might be a little worried, though. And they should be. The modern diet is feminizing men. Testosterone is important even beyond the obvious reason that it fuels our sex drive and is, in essence, what makes us male. Insufficient testosterone has been linked with an increased risk of obesity, type 2 diabetes, heart disease, low sperm count, and death.

"Both the incidence of low testosterone, or hypogonadism, in men and the annual number of testosterone prescriptions are increasing, likely as a result of the obesity epidemic and our aging population," said Frances Hayes, M.D., an endocrinologist who recently studied the connection between sugar consumption and hormones.[2] That word, *hypogonadism,* should scare you. It means that men become fatter, their testicles shrink, and their testosterone levels decrease.

Watch any televised sport and you'll see a big contributor to this problem: Every edible being advertised has been found to suppress production of testosterone and increase levels of estrogen in males. Pizza. Beer. Fast-food burgers and fries. Doughnuts and other sweets. Soda. The so-called sports drinks, which are full of sugar and salt. Even the protein supplements being sold as muscle-building aids contribute to this problem. Many of these products can contain as many calories of carbohydrates and sugar as three pieces of pie. Their cumulative impact is a massive hit to our masculinity.

The culprits that contribute to lower testosterone are the usual nutritional offenders: carbs and sugar. Research has shown that sugar consumption can lower testosterone. The authors of one scientific study found that men who drank a glucose solution experienced decreased blood levels of testosterone by as much as 25 percent, regardless of whether they had a preexisting condition such as diabetes or pre-diabetes. Free radicals induced by sugar consumption may also have a hand in lowering testosterone.[3]

Grain-based foods also depress testosterone levels, because they add to our fat stores. High insulin and low testosterone go hand in hand.[4]

Body fat itself plays a role in the loss of testosterone, as well. It converts testosterone into the female sex hormone, estrogen. The process is called "aromatizing." While men need some estrogen (just as women need some testosterone), too much estrogen in the male body is not a good thing.

It's not just excess body fat that causes some men to develop enlarged breasts—it's the overload of female hormones that are the result of a poor diet. There are obese men walking around with more estrogen than their wives.

Young men today also get too many of their daily calories from alcohol. I've seen studies that report that college-age men get as much as one-quarter of their calories from drinking. Alcohol itself lowers testosterone, but its negative effects go beyond that. The ethanol contained in alcoholic beverages causes the same spike in blood glucose and insulin resistance as any other empty calories do. The usual bad cascade results—alcohol promotes the storage of fat, and then the fat changes the testosterone into estrogen. Lacking vitamin A and other nutrients, there is nothing to block or limit this conversion.[5]

Finally, alcohol promotes inflammation, which worsens your insulin resistance. Ethanol is toxic to all the nerves in the body. So, in addition to losing their masculinity, heavy drinkers lose their brains, too.

Sadly, there will soon be fewer real males around if American men continue to eat as the commercials shown during sporting events suggest they should. These guys will still watch athletics, but they may stop taking part in them. They'll decide that sports are a little too violent, or that the physical exertion is just too difficult. This could be the end of Sunday afternoon as we know it.

CHAPTER 7

The Metaphysics Behind the Diet

First came my boyhood passion for sports and strength. Next was my immersion in the world of nutritional science and metabolism because of my wife's and son's diabetes. The third and final element that connects all the dots and accounts for my fascination with the subject of this book: The ways in which the New Evolution Diet has intersected with my intellectual life.

A little background: A great deal of my work as an economist has been in the study of complex systems, such as how natural gas prices are determined by the marketplace throughout North America. Not surprisingly, given that I had grown up in Southern California and taught at a university there, I eventually turned my attention to a notoriously murky, seemingly impossible-to-forecast industry: Hollywood.

Since its inception, the people running the motion picture business have tried to unlock the mystery of which decisions lead to financial success and which to failure. At some point, all the wisdom had been boiled down to this rueful admission by screenwriter William Goldman: "Nobody knows anything." That's exactly the kind of axiom that an economist cannot let stand untested. And so in 1995 David Walls and I gathered box office revenue data on 300 Hollywood films and began to investigate what separated the winners from the losers.

This research produced a book, *Hollywood Economics,* and several scholarly papers, but the gist is this: Goldman was right. There is no way at the outset to plan a movie's success. Neither the choice of stars or directors or writers nor the genre of movie nor the subject matter were found to make a reliable difference in how the films performed. Some big-budget movies soared at the box office, and others tanked. Small, "quality" movies made for modest sums exhibited the same range of possibilities (although with smaller stakes, of course). Neither did critical acclaim or scorn seem to matter. The sole predictive factor of a movie's future revenue was how well the movie had done since it opened: Popular movies tended to grow in popularity, as positive word of mouth attracted more filmgoers to the theater. Unpopular films fell into even deeper disfavor among audiences, and their receipts decreased.

Meanwhile, my ad hoc study of health, nutrition, and fitness continued to deepen. I had already begun to discover that our ancestors' lifestyle from 40,000 years ago could teach us how to live today. Now I was also beginning to perceive the full complexity of the systems and dynamics that determine whether or not we will be healthy.

At some point I realized that a human being is just another economic system. Indeed, your body contains an entire economy. There is the allocation of assets according to a hierarchy of needs. There are competing interests that sometimes struggle over resources and other times cooperate for the common good. There are surpluses. There are shortages. Like economies—like the movie industry—your body is a complex, decentralized system poised between chaos and order, a constantly changing situation that is, second by second, atom by atom, also adapting to those changes.

All of this runs counter to the popular illusion that what happens inside our bodies is a stable, linear, orderly process controlled by the head office—the brain—which dictates the proper actions of everything below. Far from it. You are made up of electrical, chemical, and mechanical components all under the influence of regulatory processes that try to establish equilibrium but never quite succeed. Your pancreatic cells don't take orders from your brain, your blood, or anything else except the DNA that created them. And the same is true for all the billions of cells inside you.

In the movie business, word-of-mouth reviews, more than anything, were what prompted fans to see one film instead of another, or no film at all. It is a powerful feedback loop made up of millions of small parts, each acting independently. This system has grown exponentially since the advent of the Internet. Where once millions of moviegoers chattered, now there are billions, perpetually in contact with one another, weighing in, arguing, linking, connecting and disconnecting, uploading and downloading.

It mimics perfectly what goes on inside our bodies. Billions of cells, all connected but working autonomously, with no central authority to guide them, take in information (in the form of nutrients, hormones, and so on), react, then talk back and forth at the speed of electrons, each one responding in small ways that collectively add up to a powerful force.

"Information cascade" is a term from economics to describe how even a small piece of knowledge can be amplified as it spreads from one decision maker to another. Your body is also controlled by cascades of information—your bloodstream is hit with a dose of carbohydrate, which is the signal for your pancreas to release insulin, which turns off fat burning and silences the signal from leptin, the hormone that would ordinarily tell your body that it has adequate reserves of energy and need not store any more.

Likewise, in the aging cascade, we lose metabolic fitness. And as a result, insulin rises and we grow more acidic, which further decreases metabolic health, and each event amplifies the momentum of what preceded it.

Hollywood wanted to believe that there was some stable, easy-to-predict dynamic that ruled the movie business. If there were, decisions could be made and investments taken with confidence in their outcome. Similarly, health experts used oversimplified analogies—

automobile engines and furnaces are two that come to mind—to predict how your metabolism managed nutrition and weight. All you
have to do is burn more fuel than you take in, we were instructed,
and you will reliably lose weight. Burn precisely as much as you consume and you will maintain. Burn less and you'll gain. Simple
arithmetic.

This was more a failing of human imagination than anything else.
We tend to simplify what otherwise seems overwhelmingly complicated.
But as we now know, our metabolic function is infinitely more complex
than that of a car engine or a furnace. I found myself using concepts
from other scientific disciplines to help me understand and explain the
human body's inner workings. Certainly, it is possible to get the practical
benefits of the New Evolution Diet without getting into such esoteric ter-
ritory. But I found that it helped me, a layman, to engage with the material, to frame what I was learning, and to express it.

For instance, at around the time of my movie industry studies, the
study of chaos theory was becoming fashionable in the sciences.
According to the theory, a mathematical concept first trotted out in the
19th century, certain systems that seem to be random in fact are not—
it's just difficult for us to perceive, at the outset, all the subtle factors
that set the course and determine the outcome. In time, chaos theory
was being applied in other sciences as well—everything from earth-
quake science to economics. I found that it helped me to understand
how our bodies function.

One landmark of chaos theory is the "butterfly effect." This says that
even a very small, unseen occurrence in a far-off place can have a large
eventual impact—that if a butterfly flaps its wings in Hong Kong, the
resulting breeze can trigger a cascade of atmospheric events and cause
a hurricane in Brazil.

This can be used to explain many of our bodies' inner workings.
Here's a simple one: If you go to the gym several hours after your last

meal (so that you're on a relatively empty stomach), your body will quickly burn through whatever glycogen is in your muscles and then move on to burning fat, which is the desirable state. But if on your way to the gym you have a sports drink, one with lots of carbs (meaning anything but water), you will need to burn off the glucose first. And depending on your workout, you might never get around to burning fat at all. Same exact exercise routine, very different outcomes, all because of your choice of pre-exercise beverage.

Another scientific concept, the power law, also comes up often in my discussions of health and fitness. It is based on the Pareto principle, named for Italian economist Vilfredo Pareto. In essence, it describes the relationship between how common a factor is and how much influence it exerts. It says that the most unusual events will have the greatest impact. Pareto's study, done about a century ago, determined that 80 percent of privately held land in Italy was owned by 20 percent of the population. (The principle is also called the 80/20 rule, or the law of the vital few.) Similar power laws exist all around us.

For instance, in my study of the movie business, I learned that 90 percent of the profits come from 10 percent of the movies. And for directors, 40 percent of their lifetime revenues come from a single film. Scientists have found that 40 percent of a decade's damage due to flood will come from just one such event. The Richter law of earthquakes says that the most common quakes are small, and the rare big ones do nearly all the damage. This relationship between low frequency and high impact is found again and again, in various fields of science, business, and elsewhere.[1]

Even in our everyday lives we see power laws. A man will meet many women, for instance, but only a very few—his wife (or wives, as the case may be)—will have a lasting effect. You may work alongside many colleagues, but only a handful will have a significant impact on your career. It is the few memorable moments that count more than the drip of quotidian events.

There is a power law of exercise, too: Your least frequent, most extreme exertions will have the greatest influence on your fitness. The peak moments of a workout count far more than the amount of time you spend working out. This is why a series of 40-yard sprints at full speed benefits you more than half an hour of jogging. It's also the reason why lifting a weight heavy enough to make your heart pound and your muscles burn counts more than spending hours at the gym always in your comfort zone, never truly challenging your body. When a workout becomes an unvarying, monotonous routine, it loses its effectiveness.

Power law teaches us that the average can be meaningless and even misleading. In the movie business, many films lose money, and a few are huge hits. But if you compute the average box office receipts, you may be fooled into thinking that all films earn money—which is far from the case. In fact, it is likely that *no* film earned anything like the average sum.

Similarly, my average output of energy per week may look fairly modest. But the stretches of indolence are offset by two or three sessions of extremely intense activity, which do most to determine my well-being. Ancient hunter-gatherers spent much of their time doing little or nothing. And then, every so often, they took action that would exhaust any 21st-century gym rat. Overall, they burned twice as much energy as we do. Lions sleep most of the time, but then they make up for it by chasing down, killing, and carrying away an adult gazelle. The lion doesn't try to maintain a steady output of moderate energy. It has no need to do so.

A few of the personal trainers at my gym laugh at "cardio queens," people (women *and* men) who waste hours on the treadmill and Stair-Master, trudging away but never really pushing themselves to intensity. But many more trainers recommend the unproductive exercise of "doing cardio" because they still subscribe to the energy-in, energy-out model of body weight. By doing the same cardio workout day after day, their bodies adapt to that exact level of energy demand but nothing greater. The internal message these people send is that they don't need much fast-twitch muscle fiber, and so it atrophies, and as a result, they lose bone mass, too. They remind me of a marathoner who played on my softball team—he could run all day long but was incapable of beating the throw to first base.

I use other terms and concepts that are not normally found in fitness books. *Stochasticity,* for instance, means "randomness" or "chance." A living human leaves a "trail" of events and accomplishments that is so complex that it appears to be random. That means there is no model that can compress the information that is required to describe a lifetime. The appearance of randomness is an acknowledgment of the limits of our knowledge. So it is in markets and in life.

Then there's *fractals,* another term from mathematics, which refers to jagged lines, such as are found in an electrocardiogram. The heart has no standard beat; it is constantly being acted upon by whatever is going on within and also outside your body. And so the time intervals between beats vary constantly. If the intervals become too random, it's a problem, but it's also unhealthy if your heartbeat is too regular and metronomic. The jagged, fractal variations are evidence of your system's adaptability—your heart's ability to respond properly to stimulus. A heart that beats to a fractal pattern follows a power law distribution of the intervals between beats.[2]

My particular form of engagement with the subject of health and fitness has even proven to have a metaphysical side. Each of us has what I call an ensemble of stochastic life paths—the choices that we make. You make each choice in life based on your understanding of the possibility that it will take you where you want to be. But you don't determine the outcome, only the probabilities. Each path leads to more choices: a cascade to echo all the other cascades that rule our lives. Choosing the path is the extent of your control—beyond that, it's out of your hands. You choose, and then life rolls the dice.

For example, you can determine what you eat and drink and how you will exercise. But then your genes express themselves as they will. They are beyond your control. You can't even completely determine your genes' environment, since outside factors (such as air and water quality) and internal ones (like emotional stress) also have a say. I learned about the limits of control when caring for my first wife, Bonnie, through her terminal illness. I learned it again in my studies of the movie industry, and now in the course of my ongoing education in health.

It has even allowed me to recognize, in this thought, the Zen of the hunter-gatherer lifestyle: There is no failure, only feedback.

Sir Steven and Michael Phelps

What do Olympic rower Steve Redgrave and Olympic swimmer Michael Phelps have in common? Both of these athletes are royalty. Steve Redgrave was one of Britain's top athletes. In fact, he was given a knighthood by the Queen of England. The U.S. media and advertisers knighted Michael Phelps.

In the years 1984–2000, Steve Redgrave won five Olympic gold medals in rowing. His training was arduous and his diet atrocious. Michael Phelps won eight Olympic gold medals at the 2008 Summer Games. His training was even more arduous than Redgrave's, and his diet even worse.

Sir Steven developed type 2 diabetes by the age of 35. Michael Phelps's diet may yet lead to the same fate. Briefly reviewing the consequences of diet among great athletes is a useful application of the science that guides the principles of this book.

In a May 2005 edition of the *Daily Telegraph,* Elizabeth Grice colorfully describes Sir Steven's diet and training regime:

> Steve Redgrave's description of the body fuel he needed to get him through four training sessions a day in the run-up to his fifth consecutive Olympic gold medal is Bunterish in its amplitude, the drooling dream of any pudding-loving member of the human race who has ever grappled with a weight problem.

To keep up the phenomenal energy levels required for a typical day ploughing the water, Sir Steven needed to consume 6,000 calories, starting with a hefty four Weetabix for breakfast. Between the first two sessions on the Thames, he would down a bowl of porridge, liberally dressed with sugar, or scrambled eggs on toast and a large jug of fruit juice.

Refueling between the afternoon sessions usually meant soup, followed by a large pasta dish, pudding and another flagon of juice. Back home to toast or malted loaf—even if on the way he may have stopped for petrol and picked up a chocolate bar, a packet of wine gums and a bag of doughnuts to keep his blood sugar levels up.

For the main meal of the day, spaghetti Bolognese would ideally be followed by rice pudding or apple pie and ice cream. A bowl of cereal at bedtime and he would know he had done his bit for England. Arise, if possible, Sir Steve.

Michael Phelps reportedly consumes 12,000 calories a day, twice as many calories as Steve Redgrave did. Clemente Lisi describes Phelps's diet on the *New York Post*'s Web page (August 13, 2008) in the following way:

> Phelps' diet—which involves ingesting 4,000 calories every time he sits down for a meal—resembles that of a reckless over-eater rather than an Olympian.
>
> Phelps lends a new spin to the phrase "Breakfast of Champions" by starting off his day by eating three fried-egg sandwiches loaded with cheese, lettuce, tomatoes, fried onions and mayonnaise.
>
> He follows that up with two cups of coffee, a five-egg omelet, a bowl of grits, three slices of French toast topped with powdered sugar and three chocolate-chip pancakes.
>
> At lunch, Phelps gobbles up a pound of enriched pasta and two large ham and cheese sandwiches slathered with mayo on white

bread—capping off the meal by chugging about 1,000 calories worth of energy drinks.

For dinner, Phelps really loads up on the carbs—what he needs to give him plenty of energy for his five-hours-a-day, six-days-a-week regimen—with a pound of pasta and an entire pizza.

He washes all that down with another 1,000 calories worth of energy drinks.

Note that both reporters adhere to the fallacious energy-balance model. They argue that these athletes are protected from obesity because their energy expenditures equal or exceed their intakes. This is not necessarily so.

Athletes who consume large amounts of energy from carbohydrate sources make tremendous demands on their pancreas. The beta cells of the pancreas that sense and release glucose, and the insulin receptors that respond to insulin, wear out from repeated assaults of glucose and free radicals. Inflammation attacks and makes the cells and cell receptors less sensitive. Consequently, over time, athletes tend to require a larger release of insulin with each dose of carbohydrate they consume (as would anyone who consumes the staggering amount of carbohydrates that they do).

Refilling the muscles quickly with glycogen after exertion is completely counterproductive, because low muscle glycogen is the state that raises insulin sensitivity. Restricting carbohydrate intake following exercise enhances insulin sensitivity for at least 48 hours. It also causes the body to burn more fat as fuel.

I suspect that many athletes are setting themselves up for mitochondrial damage and the host of health problems known as metabolic syndrome. (I think this is why so many retired athletes appear in weight-loss ads.) They are flowing so much energy through oxidative metabolism pathways that their mitochondria release large amounts of free radicals. In time, these reactive oxygen species will damage the energy-producing mitochondria and reduce their output. I hope these athletes are not damaging their longevity or setting preconditions for cancer or mitochondrial decline. Reactive oxygen species (ROS) are free radicals of varying reactivity (hence, species since they vary in the damage they do) that damage cellular DNA and are among the prime promoters of cancer.

It would be easier for athletes to sustain high caloric intake if they consumed more fat and less simple carbohydrate. This would lessen the load on the digestion process, too. But some athletes still fear that without eating massive amounts of carbs, they will not replenish muscle glycogen quickly enough for the next training session. The evidence doesn't fully support that point of view. Nor does it follow that the carbs must be consumed every day to bring muscle glycogen to optimal level. The literature is appallingly weak regarding diets for athletics. And the rate of glycogen repletion following a training session has never been made clear.

This much we *do* know: A low-carb diet leads to a reduction in athletic performance. That is the consensus view and has been shown in a long line of studies. However, none of these studies allowed a sufficient period of adaptation by the athlete to the diet. It takes weeks to adjust to a low-carbohydrate diet, and none of the studies allowed sufficient time for that. So in my opinion, the question remains open.

On the other hand, the consequence of excessive carbohydrate consumption, even among active athletes, is not in question. It is eventually ruinous to their health.

Contemporary hunter-gatherers have legendary endurance even though they eat little carbohydrate and certainly do not carb-load before an event the way modern athletes do. It is estimated that members of the previously mentioned Aché tribe of Paraguay expend 4,000 to 5,000 calories a day foraging, with meat and fat as their primary fuels (they also eat high-energy tubers that make a small contribution to their intake). The Inuit diet consists of fat and protein with almost no carbohydrate. They hunt and fish in cold, difficult terrain with ease. And Native Americans historically relied on pemmican as their fuel, a mixture of meat, fat, and berries. They could live for days on the energy, protein, and antioxidants it supplied.

Doctor Stephen Phinney tested endurance and peak aerobic power of subjects after a 6-week period on a low-carbohydrate, moderate-protein, moderate-fat, very low-calorie diet, while making sure they had adequate sodium and potassium intake.[1]

The average subject lost over 20 pounds in 6 weeks. Their peak aerobic power did not decline—a fact that suggests that their muscles were not depleted of glycogen, their primary fuel for performance. Endurance declined initially but then increased to a higher level than baseline at the end of 6 weeks. All this occurred on a diet that supplied fewer calories than the subjects expended.

In a second study, of bicycle racers, Phinney prepared the subjects for 1 week on their standard diet, in which 67 percent of energy came from carbohydrate.[2] This was followed by 4 weeks on the Inuit diet, consisting of 83 percent of energy as fat, 15 percent as protein, and 2 percent as carbohydrate. To maintain mineral balance during the adjustment period, the subjects were given 1.5 grams of potassium, 3 grams of sodium, 600 milligrams of calcium, 300 milligrams of magnesium, and a standard multivitamin.

The bicyclists noted a modest decline in energy during the first week of the Inuit diet, but after that their endurance returned to baseline. There was a 2 percent decline in the first 2 weeks in sprint performance, due to declining muscle glycogen. By week 6, though, maximum oxygen expenditure (VO^2 max) returned to baseline and endurance time increased slightly. The subjects were using fat, not carbs, to fuel their activity. Consistent results have been found in animal studies that show adequate glycogen repletion and endurance performance of rats on a high-fat diet.

I am not arguing in favor of a high-fat diet—the philosophy I am advocating is moderate fat. But I would like to point out that the current research does not support the necessity of a high-carbohydrate diet unequivocally and that the health hazards of high-carbohydrate intake and extreme exercise are real and serious.

When training ceases, the visceral adipose tissue (VAT) is no longer kept in check and begins to accumulate more fat. Sumo wrestlers are fat but have small VAT deposits because their intense training limits its mass. When the sport is over, the VAT gains size and begins to sabotage metabolism. Insulin sensitivity, therefore, declines as the VAT tissues secrete hormones and cytokines that promote insulin resistance and inflammation. This, I think, is why so many ex-athletes gain weight and develop metabolic syndrome.

With the cessation of hard training, and the dietary habits developed over years of training, weight management becomes a problem for the inactive athlete. Because the brain is now resistant to the action of insulin, thanks to years of high-carbohydrate abuse, it lives on the edge of glucose starvation. Retired athletes will find that they "need" glucose or starch to avoid feeling edgy and tired. They will feel the need to return to old foods and eating habits, which are hard to resist: Ingesting large amounts of carbs triggers a burst of free radicals that damage the appetite control cells of the brain.

All human brains are biased toward excess energy intake and low energy expenditure, as we discussed in the introduction. This is the lazy overeater evolutionary adaptation. Consequently, many former athletes find it difficult not to overeat, and carbs are their primary vice. Most former professional athletes gain weight and many develop diabetes.

CHAPTER 8

The Competition Within

It may be true that once you start to look for evidence of Darwinism, you find it everywhere. But it is also undeniable that inside of us, as outside, exists a fierce competition for survival. Outside, there is the struggle over resources, and only those with the genes best adapted to thrive in their environment will do so. One bird's beak is just marginally better equipped to get at its food source, and its shorter-beaked neighbor exits the stage for good. Inside, there are similar battles for dominance being fought. There are even good guys and bad guys, since the winner will often determine the state of our health. Here are three of the key contests going on inside you even as you read these words.

1. Your Brain versus Your Pancreas

Or, to be more precise, your brain versus insulin.

The following explanation is kind of tricky because it involves one of the complex hormonal cascades that characterize the metabolic process. At some point it will seem as though insulin is the bad guy in this battle, but it's not the hormone's fault. Blame the magic of modern food engineering.

Now then, let's start at the top. Your brain primarily runs on glucose. (In truth, the organ can also use two other substances as fuel—ketones and lactate—but glucose is the main course.) The demand for glucose is almost constant, since your brain will die if it goes more than a few minutes without it. When your brain needs a hit, it broadcasts the message: Send glucose. Your liver responds first, releasing glucose it has saved for just this occasion into the bloodstream. Your muscles also contain amino acids that the liver can turn into glucose. Your fat cells, too, release energy they've stored which can be turned into glucose in the liver or can be metabolized to produce ketones, which the brain can use to offset its need for glucose.

And that would be enough to feed even an organ as greedy as the human brain—except that your pancreas has its own response to all that glucose in the bloodstream: It releases insulin. Now, some insulin is necessary at this point, because without it, your tissues can't access glucose. But if too much insulin is released, it sets off a series of unfortunate events, and the modern diet may have conditioned your pancreas to do precisely that.

This means trouble because insulin has its own marching orders: Store glucose in muscle and fat; pull it right out of the bloodstream. Which is what happens to all that glucose that's been released, meaning that not enough of it has reached your brain. Still starved and now truly impatient, the brain sends your body another message: *Eat!* Your brain is worried because, as far as it knows, glucose is still a scarce nutrient, as it was 40,000 years ago. Even a little delay makes your brain concerned about survival. Of course, you don't know why your brain seems so frantic. But you do get the urgent message: *Eat something!* So off you run to the kitchen to do just that, and then your pancreas notices and releases even more insulin. Which stores more fat. Which causes your brain to demand another feeding. And so it goes, around and around. You can see how a person might become overweight.

Here's a good question: Why would evolution, which has mostly enabled us to survive over millions of years, allow such a faulty and dangerous system to prevail? Well, keep in mind that many millennia ago there were no foods capable of triggering a massive insulin release, like our modern groceries are. The brain was well fed back then precisely because there was no grain, no simple carbs, and no pizza or Wonder Bread or Twinkies to send your insulin soaring and then crashing. A typical kitchen today probably contains more glucose or glucose-elevating foods than our ancestors saw in a lifetime. The cereal section of the supermarket may be one of the most dangerous places your children can play.

Who Should Win: Your brain.

What to Do About It: Your liver, muscles, and fat are actually capable of supplying enough glucose to keep the brain well fed without help from external sources, like carbs. Without this capability, the human species would not have survived. But in order for this mechanism to work properly, you need to lay off bread, baked goods, sugar, and grains. Give it a try.

2. Your Muscle versus Your Fat

Most people have a simplistic understanding of the role of muscle and fat: Muscle is there so our bodies can move and do things and look good, we believe, and fat is there . . . well, why *is* fat there? We have the general sense that some of it is needed for "padding" (as though you were a sofa), but beyond that we see it as a hindrance, a nuisance, a bad thing.

Both conceptions are wrong, of course.

Metabolically speaking, fat and muscle are highly active tissue. The fat we eat is a form of nutrient, one of the three we require, the other two being protein and carbohydrate. The fat we store is necessary as a supply of energy, on which our muscles draw continually as the need arises and then release either ketones or lactate that can fuel the brain. The brain uses all these fuels: glucose, ketones, and lactate. Fat wouldn't exist if there were no good reason for it to do so. But if we all ate as we did 100,000 years ago, we would store just enough of it to provide energy and not much more. In fact, the challenge would be to build up *enough* fat for times of food scarcity.[1]

But as we know by now, contemporary eating habits mislead our bodies into storing far more energy than we require. It's worth noting that if your body fat drops too low, you will die. But there seems to be no data on the upper limit of how much extra fat a person can have and still go on living. Once-shocking reports of 700- to 1,000-pound-plus individuals have now become less sensational.[2]

Fat crosses the line and becomes hazardous to health when it constitutes too high a percentage of our total body weight. This question of body composition is central to good health. In my opinion, you should be around 11 percent fat if you are a male, 18 percent if you are a female. Anything higher than that is above the evolutionary norm and begins to alter your metabolism.[3] Even though the NIH says healthy body fat levels are 20–21 percent for women and 13–17 percent for men, this is another area where my own numbers are far superior to the "norm" and more like our ancestors or modern athletes for whom the standard was closer to 5–13 percent for men (mine is 6.7 percent right now) and 12–22 percent for women.

Fat damages your metabolism by releasing fatty acids that can be beneficial in healthy amounts but harmful in excess. The amount that is secreted is proportional to the amount of body fat—the more overweight you are, the more harmful substances (including cholesterol, steroid hormones, prostaglandins, retinol, and inflammatory cytokines such as tumor necrosis factor-alpha and interleukin-6) your fat releases. Cells in your body are continually dying and being replaced by new ones. That's nature at work. But when fat cells die, they release oxidized fatty acids; the oxidation is the result of your immune system attacking and inflaming the cells and their contents. Someone who is very overweight has a lot of fat cells and, therefore, a lot of cells dying and releasing their damaged contents, which inflame other bodily tissues.[4]

When fat stores become large, they also release hormones such as leptin, vascular growth factor, angiotensin, and some proteins of the immune system. The inflammatory factors secreted by fat contribute to premature aging and make you resistant to insulin, prompting your body to produce too much of it for your own good. When that happens, your muscle and brain get less of the energy they need, since more of it goes into fat. That's the insidious thing about the process—fat wants to create more fat.

In addition to all that, abdominal (visceral) fat physically intrudes into the space meant for your organs, muscles, and blood vessels until it impedes them from doing their jobs properly. So you see, fat isn't merely sitting there, ugly but otherwise inert. It is an active hazard to your health. Fat could even be considered a kind of tumor; because its growth is unchecked, it steals nutrients from other cells, and is attacked by the immune system.[5]

Muscle, too, does more than is apparent to the casual observer. Of course, it has its structural and mechanical tasks to fulfill. But it's not a stretch to say that muscle actually acts as medicine.

The role of muscle, like that of fat, is also determined by the size of its presence—have enough muscle and it helps maintain overall good health; have too little and it puts your health in danger.

Muscle supplies amino acids so that your immune system can build killer cells. Muscle is also the disposal site for glucose. The tissue burns energy continuously. This means that when you have adequate muscle, you can eat plenty and not gain weight.

Muscle also helps to fuel your brain. It contains amino acids the liver uses to make glucose for the brain to use, meaning you will need to consume less glucose in your diet.

Finally, muscle gives you the physical capacity to do things, so you will be more active. Muscle allows you ease of movement. And it supports your skeletal system so that you will not lose bone mass as you age.[6]

Who Should Win: Muscle, of course.

What to Do About It: Increase and maintain your muscle by challenging it on a regular basis, which means you need to move it against the stress of resistance. For most of us, that will require some time at the gym, lifting weights. You also must feed your muscle tissue with sufficient protein to fuel its growth. Rest it, too, so the muscle can restore itself.

3. Good Stress versus Bad Stress

The word *stress* has taken on a solely negative connotation today, although without stress of any kind we would be unrecognizable even to ourselves. We have lived with it since day one—the universe was created by stress, and stress has played a part in every moment since. But there is good stress and there is bad, and while the latter is inescapable, we can minimize it while maximizing the former.

Good stress is the physical kind. For our purposes, it is self-imposed activity—exercise of one form or another. It could be weight lifting, playing tennis, or a sprint uphill. It is acute, meaning it lasts for short, well-defined periods of time. Our endocrine systems experience our physical activity in the same way those of hunter-gatherers felt their exertion as they went about their daily routine. We release certain hormones in response to acute stress—mainly adrenaline—that get us through the event quickly. Our ancient ancestors' emergencies also tended to be of the short-duration variety, the kind that the fight-or-flight instinct was designed to handle.

Acute, meaning short-term, stress is good because it triggers an adaptive response that makes us resistant to all types of stress, not just the physical variety. Our antioxidant defenses are strengthened when we exercise. Our hearts grow stronger and our blood vessels more flexible. Our nervous systems shift toward a more peaceful state.

But if the stress lasts longer, other hormones are released—cortisol, mostly, which is an essential hormone that keeps us alive, except when it is released in a chronic fashion. When that happens, and we are exposed to cortisol for too long, it actually costs us neurons in the brain, muscle, and bone. Cortisol makes us gain weight because it causes insulin resistance. Too much of this hormone damages the nerves, too. And unlike our ancient ancestors, we have lots of long-duration stresses, mostly of the emotional and psychological kind. Money woes, job worries, relationship problems, difficulties with health—these are the kinds of stress that fight-or-flight can't resolve, and so the stress becomes chronic. As with diet, evolution hasn't done such a great job of anticipating the way we live today.

Who Should Win: Acute stress of short duration.

What to Do About It: Exercise. Move your body in a way that will bring you joy. Beyond that, you need to find a way to relieve or even dispel all the chronic stresses that are doing you no good.

CHAPTER 9

Age Like Me

Caged lab animals live about three times longer than their wild relatives. We modern humans live about three times longer than our wild ancestors, almost 90 years versus about 31 for them.

But our prehistoric forebears remained healthy, fit, lean, and strong right to the end. They retained their vitality into "old" age because they were active and ate only natural foods (not that they had much choice in either regard).

We outlive them not because we are superior in any way. It's just that we in developed countries don't have to worry about starvation, predation, infection, exposure, drought, and all the other potentially fatal threats to survival that civilization has tamed, if not eradicated.

Of course, we have plenty else to worry about. Inactivity, starchy foods, and obesity lead to a loss of insulin sensitivity and a host of hormonal changes that accelerate the aging process. We live longer than our ancestors did, but we spend a higher proportion of our lives in disability.

Your lean body mass makes the difference between aging well and aging badly. It's the "active you"—the engine that carries you through life. It's the store of protein on which your immune system relies to destroy pathogens. It's the measure of your organ mass and function.

The rate of loss of lean body mass is so powerful a predictor of health status that it seems to be part of the process of dying. If you were to lose 40 percent of your lean body mass, you would not survive. Degenerative, lethal diseases like AIDS, sepsis, and others cause a wasting of lean body tissue. Sufferers die when their body mass declines that 40 percent.

But rapid protein wastage is a cause, not just an indicator, of death. What we call "normal" aging is in reality the long-term effect of sedentary living combined with carbohydrate abuse. It's the accumulation of damage from too little exertion and too much insulin.

After we enter our thirties, we lose lean body mass at a rate between 2 and 5 percent per decade. There are large individual differences, however, that depend on diet and lifestyle: for example, I have lost none of my lean body mass. Most of the muscle we lose is fast-twitch fiber, because we no longer challenge our bodies sufficiently. As we settle into old age, we also lose bone density, making us vulnerable to damaging falls since our muscles are not strong or quick enough to keep us upright.[1]

Centenarians tend to have low fasting insulin and are strong. They are not fat. I love the story about a woman who died at the age of 115 after falling off a ladder. She must have been strong. She probably had very low insulin, given that she was thin enough to climb high enough to sustain a fatal fall. Low insulin with low fat is a self-reinforcing feedback loop; each fosters the other. Centenarians evidently have reached a metabolic state that turns down the aging cascade. Insulin resistance and physical strength are excellent predictors of expected life span past the age of 35, and they become more important with each advancing year.[2] Leg and grip strength are strong predictors of long-term health.

Finally, inflammation plays an important role in determining how well (or how badly) you age. Inflammation is a product of your body's protective response against unknown intruders—irritants or pathogens. It is intended to remove the intruder and heal any damage it has caused. But persistent immune system attacks on damaged sites harm the cells nearby, resulting in prolonged or chronic inflammation.

As we saw in Chapter 2, your C-reactive protein level, normally tested in a metabolic panel, is one reliable measure of inflammation. High levels are predictive of atherosclerosis and heart disease. A great deal of inflammation can result from poor diet and insufficient activity.

If you know how strong someone is, what their insulin level is, and how inflamed they are, you know quite a lot about how long they can expect to live. You can also predict with a high degree of accuracy how long that person will be free of chronic disease and how much time (if any) they will spend in a nursing home. The occupants of nursing homes typically have elevated insulin levels, low strength, and high levels of inflammation. They age badly. You can do better.

Life is an event-counting process, and some events count more than others. Traumas such as injuries, financial or emotional difficulties, and deaths of loved ones all weigh heavily on us. So the first steps to ensure a healthy old age need to be taken while you are still young: Get a good education, save your money, and don't take unnecessary risks. (Of course the best longevity-related advice of all is not within your control: Be born with good genes.)

Some debilitating life events are well within your control, however, such as the number of diet-related insulin or glucose spikes that will affect your body and brain over the years. Each one of these events lessens insulin sensitivity and kills neurons. Cells are damaged, and they can take only so much of that before they commit the equivalent of cell suicide—they execute their built-in death program for the sake of their neighboring cells and the survival of the organism itself (you).

Many elderly are poorly nourished. They have little interest in food, or not much of an appetite, and do not prepare fresh, nutritious meals. In some cases, their income or their health prevents them from eating nutritious foods. As a result, they lack key vitamins and, more seriously, protein in their diets. They are unable to retain muscle mass, which encourages them to overeat—their brains sense the lack of protein and seek to obtain it from food. As a result, they just eat *more* bad foods, taking in too much energy and too little nutrition.

Beyond getting adequate protein, the elderly should include ample servings of vegetables and fruits in their diets to reduce the acidity of their bodies. Aging seems to advance the body toward a more acidic state, which increases the damage done by free radicals and also promotes loss of skeletal mass.

Fortunately, it is simple to avoid the highly acidic state that seems to go hand in hand with aging. Eliminating grains from your diet is one way to do this, as grains and foods made from grains are acidic. Vegetables and fruits, on the other hand, are alkaline and tend to neutralize the acids produced by eating grains or exercising. (Unfortunately, exercising does promote the acidic state as a side effect.) Taking a potassium bicarbonate supplement is another effective way to neutralize acid.

What you *don't* eat also matters. I hesitate to suggest to older readers that they eat less, since that might mean eating less protein. But current research in aging and life extension supports the connection between nutrient availability and gene expression. And so even the elderly may benefit from occasional fasting and glucose restriction.

As discussed in Chapter 4, some people practice calorie restriction (CR) as a means of trying to extend life expectancy. People who practice CR limit their intake to as little as 900 to 1,000 calories daily, meaning they live in a state of constant hunger. Those who can tolerate this perpetual misery seem to show good biomarkers in tests, but they lose a good deal of muscle mass as the body adjusts its composition to their energy intake to maintain the constant energy needs of the brain and metabolically active tissues. On the whole, they have less muscle and a bit more fat than they would have if they ate more.

However, other research now seems to point the finger at glucose rather than total calorie intake as the aging culprit. If this proves to be true, then the people who practice calorie restriction may be starving themselves unnecessarily. And cutting glucose intake would certainly be a lot easier to live with than feeling constant hunger. This is why glucose restriction, rather than calorie restriction, is one of the pillars of the New Evolution Diet.

Glucose restriction also may be beneficial to mitochondrial function. The mitochondria are the energy furnaces inside our cells that process glucose and fat to produce ATP (adenosine triphosphate), the universal fuel within the body. The number and functioning of the mitochondria determine the amount of energy that is available to the cell. Mitochondrial DNA is affected by too-high levels of blood glucose. Even just a few days of exposure to high glucose may result in the accumulation of oxidized proteins and reduced expression of mitochondrial DNA. On the other hand, glucose restriction improves DNA repair.

Here's why it works: Our genes have their own priorities, with number one being their own propagation. They have no particular feelings about whether we as human beings survive; they are in it for themselves. They don't keep track of our years, but they do receive information about us from the nutrients they receive, and they base their actions on what they learn. If they get plenty of glucose from the carbohydrates in our diet, they intuit that there is abundant energy out there. Based on that message, they feel confident that the environment can sustain lots of our offspring. And so our genes feel no particular pressure to repair themselves.

Low glucose sends the opposite message: Your genes can't rely on your reproductive prowess, and so they need to maintain their own health. That's precisely the message we want them to receive, even if to do so we have to trick them by cutting out carbs.

We can also send that message by burning fat instead of glucose. When bacteria are fed glycerol (the backbone of fat molecules), they live as long as they do when they are denied calories through chronic caloric restriction. It appears that when the body has only fat to burn instead of glucose, it is a signal to genes that nutrition is scarce. And so they must keep themselves in good repair.

A lean, muscular body promotes low insulin levels. I am aging at a slow rate in part because my insulin is low.[3] Low body fat also guarantees low blood fats, most of which come from a person's own abdominal fat rather than from diet. But it is body composition, not just body fat, that is the issue; you must have the right balance of muscle to fat to promote the hormone drives that keep you young and your brain well balanced and nourished.

Your muscle is also part of your immune system. It functions as a reservoir of protein to proliferate killer cells when they are needed in your body's defense.

Exercise also offers antiaging benefits. Intermittent, intense, and brief workouts build muscle mass that burns energy continuously. This type of exercise promotes hormone drives that keep you young and change the body's metabolic pathways so that the energy you consume feeds muscle and organ mass, not fat. Remember that the intensity of your exercise regimen is also important, as intense activity engages the fast-twitch fibers of your muscles, which are the key to staying young. Retaining your metabolic headroom through intense, brief, and variable training promotes your overall health and vitality. If there is a fountain of youth to be found at the gym, it is strength training. Weight lifting silences or reduces the expression of at least 30 genes that promote aging.[4] It produces an acute use of energy restriction and, therefore, mimics the effect of calorie restriction. Individuals as old as 90 respond well to weight training and many can double their strength within a few months of regular exercise. Most of the benefits of strength training can be attained in one brief (no more than 15 minutes), safe, and somewhat intense session per week. I would suggest two even-briefer sessions weekly so that insulin sensitivity and sleep are enhanced by your exertions.

Aging is a process of accumulated damage. Much of our internal rust comes from oxygen. We've discussed this elsewhere in the book: We need oxygen to live, but it is a double-edged sword, for it also gradually kills us. Oxygenation fosters harmful free radicals, or ROS, which attack healthy cells by stealing their electrons and promoting inflammation and cell death.

A diet high in antioxidants, either from plant-based foods or supplements, decreases the oxygenation of cells and, therefore, combats aging. In addition, a low-glucose diet suppresses free radicals.[5] It also limits the formation of glucose protein molecules, glycosylated protein, and advanced glycation end products, which link together cells and tissues. Here's why that linkage is bad for you: When your body combines ROS and sugar, it forms a glue that attaches proteins to one another and makes us stiff and brittle.

The acidity of a grain-based diet is another contributor to unhealthy aging. The more acid in our bodies, the more inflamed we become. In turn, inflammation and obesity promote insulin resistance, which leads to more insulin, and the feedback loop becomes self-reinforcing. My diet eliminates grains, beans, legumes, and milk, which cause acidification, and offers the plant polyphenols and other compounds that reduce inflammation.

All in all, my own experience with aging has been a good one. By the numbers, I'm actually better off now than I was in my younger days. My insulin levels have gone down over the years as I've adjusted my diet and begun intermittent fasting.[6] My good cholesterol has risen, and my bad cholesterol has fallen, along with my triglycerides and blood glucose. My blood pressure is where it should be. My doctor tells me he's never seen a testosterone level as high as mine.

Back in 1995, when I was 58, I had a test of so-called biological age done at the Colgan Institute in California. As I scan the list of "biomarkers of aging," I see readings of a biological age of 29 years for cholesterol,

30 for blood pressure, 34 for glucose, 19 for body fat, 22 for reaction speed, and 23 for grip strength. My overall biological age at the time was shown to be 31. Even if you have some skepticism for ratings such as this (as I do), it does show that I have young blood, which is a good thing. Of course, I had a foundation of strength dating back to my youth, and I have trained hard in the gym and remained active and health conscious ever since.

Adulthood has not been without its challenges, naturally. One of these was a more or less constant inflammation. The other was chronic lower back pain. The inflammation was due in part to a lack of antioxidants in my diet. Some changes in my eating habits—increased fruits and vegetables, plus some antioxidant supplements—have fixed that, to a degree.

I was tested for rheumatoid arthritis because I had been suffering with the connective tissue form of arthritis. I think this was from swinging a heavy bat in my baseball and softball days, when I had been a real home run hitter. It left my wrist ligaments vulnerable to inflammation. I was also working out incorrectly, doing too many bodybuilder exercises and too many repetitions. Once I switched to my new style of workouts and began eating better and taking antioxidants, the problem began to resolve itself. Yet even then it never quite went away until I stopped drinking beer.

I loved beer, partly because I drink huge amounts of liquid. Back then I drank up to four beers a day. But I would notice that my face reddened when I drank, a sign of inflammation. This is a clear symptom that you are allergic to whatever it is you're consuming. The almost paradoxical thing is that an allergen prompts a stress response that releases adrenaline, which in turn gives you a little bit of a high. It's just one more reason you become slightly addicted to things that are bad for you. I think this is why some people say they can never give up bread, or pasta, or pizza: The hormonal response to the inflammation caused by eating grains feels too good to stop.

The back pain was to be expected. I had injured my lower back while racing motorcycles, and my mother also had back and neck pain. It's especially common among those who have been as athletic as I was. From baseball I turned to academia, meaning I was spending too much time sitting at desks, reading and writing, another cause of back pain.

My solution was to stop doing all the static stretching exercises that had been recommended to cure my back pain. Instead, I focused on the abdominal brace stance (as described in Chapter 5). This way of standing and carrying myself caused me to focus on tilting my pelvis to restore the proper curve in my lower back, and to lift my chin and heart. When I worked out, I also made sure to adequately stretch my hamstrings, which is another way to correct pelvis alignment.

All these changes helped. When I was about 64, a year before I retired from UC Irvine, I was in the most muscular and "ripped" state of my life at 208 pounds. One day I was Rollerblading along the walk at Newport Beach, no shirt, just shorts and the skates. I rolled through a little opening between four young women walking alongside one another. As I passed them, one of them pretended to start chasing me. I loved it—she must have been about 18 and had no idea I was old enough to be her grandfather.

A few years later, playing softball, I hit an over-the-fence home run and later made a diving catch in the outfield. When I came up to bat next time, the catcher told the umpire to give me a saliva test for steroids and to check my age on my driver's license. In my last game in slow-pitch softball (I was 71 at the time), I hit three home runs over the fence. I would say that my health has steadily improved over the past three decades. I have none of the old aches and pains. And, having maintained my good health, I think I have acquired a kind of wisdom. It's a love of learning and a perspective that come from having abundant energy. I truly feel fearless because, by now, I know I can handle whatever life throws at me.

I can say that because just a few years back, a lot was thrown at me. My first wife, Bonnie, developed what is called systemic vasculitis. This is a terrible disease in which the autoimmune system attacks the small blood vessels, causing them to disintegrate and collapse. This causes the body's microcirculation to decline, stealing nutrients and failing to deliver oxygen to the cells. She began to waste away, body and brain. Over the course of 2 years she was dying, slowly. My mother, who lived near us, was in declining health then also.

During the last year of Bonnie's decline, I had almost no sleep. It is an odd thing about people who are dying; they sleep during the day because they fear the night. I think illness makes the mind retreat into more primitive regions, where the dark of night still equals danger. To cope with the strain of losing my lifelong companion, I deliberately ate less, episodically, in order to trigger my stress resistance. I dropped about 10 pounds, to a low, for me, of 195.

Bonnie's bravery still inspires me. She kept her great sense of humor almost to the end, until the fear took even that. She often told me that she was unhappy at the thought of dying before my mother did. She felt that a wife should always outlive her mother-in-law. Well, she made it. Bonnie died on January 22, 2006. My mother, Ella De Vany, passed away on January 21.

I got through this difficult time thanks to the belief that I did not have the power to save my wife, nor did medicine. In fact, her disease was so rare there were no doctors capable of treating it. Out of this tragedy came my attitude that I have only one moment of power, which is now, and that I can determine not the outcome but only the probable path.

I had to find a new life that did not revolve around caring for my wife. I was still in terrific health and felt I could do anything I wanted. I briefly considered running "barefoot through the condos" and dating women of all ages. But I thought better of it. At 70, I did not want to raise another child.

My neighbor at the time was a nurse. She stopped by to see me often as I sat in the hospital, waiting to visit Bonnie. Six months or so after Bonnie's death, her husband asked me if I wanted to meet a friend of theirs who also worked at the hospital. I'm glad I said yes, because she turned out to be the woman I would marry. Once I met her, I had no interest in dating any others. She was close to my age,

trim, full of life, and funny as all heck. And even though she is a phenomenal cook in her own right, she even allowed me to prepare the
meals we shared in my empty house. We dated regularly and laughed
a lot. I think I fell in love the third time I saw her.

We went to Italy together so I could ride motorcycles on the isle of
Elba, where I proposed to her on the beach. We've been married for 3
years now. Her health was good when we met, but her doctor had been
alarmed at her less-than-stellar metabolic panel, and her blood pressure
was high. All these issues quickly resolved themselves when she began
to eat and exercise as I did. She even lost five dress sizes in a few
months. Not a bad way to grow old together.

My Supplements

Eating well is crucial to maintaining good health, of course, but it's not always enough. That said, I find that dietary supplements are limited in their effectiveness, so my supplement regimen is minimalistic and inexpensive. My focus is to maintain lean body mass, excellent insulin sensitivity, and high immune function; to promote good mood; and to reduce inflammation. I do think that supplements are partly responsible for the fact that I have not had so much as a head cold in more than 25 years. I am never sick (knock on wood).

My two main supplements provide amino acids and antioxidants. These are critical for several reasons. Good mood and high immune function are intimately connected to adequate intake of amino acids. This is especially important for women, as serotonin levels are sometimes lower in females than in males. This is due, in part, to low levels of amino acids—which are necessary for neurotransmitter synthesis—in their diets. I think one reason women are more prone to depression than men is because they typically eat less animal protein.

Amino acids also assist the immune system. Muscle and diet are the primary sources of amino acids for the immune system to draw on when it must gear up to fight an infection.

Inflammation is a systemic problem that reduces insulin sensitivity and damages every tissue in the body. While the fruits and vegetables in my diet provide substantial amounts of antioxidants, I also take a sophisticated product that provides the master antioxidant, glutathione. I have taken it for more than 25 years.

Here's what I take and why:

- **Vitamin D:** 1,000 international units (IU) each day, up to 5,000 units on cloudy days or when I can't get outside in the sunlight. I get outside in sunlight most days, exposing my arms, face, and legs on the tennis court or just walking, meaning I get plenty of vitamin D the natural way. I may sit out by the pool or in my backyard without a shirt for a few minutes, too. About an hour of full sunshine can equal as much as 40,000 units of vitamin D, which is all you need. But many people don't spend enough time outdoors, and so they should take a supplement. Children are particularly vulnerable to vitamin D deficiency, especially kids who spend too much time indoors. Milk is not a good source of vitamin D and, in fact, most of it is added after the milk is processed. (Besides, beyond the age of 3, children should not drink milk. It is highly allergenic and actually increases stomach acidity, which depletes minerals in the bones. Cow's milk has many problems, unless you're a calf.)

- **Omega-3 fish oil capsules:** 1,000 milligrams with each meal when I do not eat fish. I make sure to take this supplement when I eat beef or pork, to offset the high saturated fat content. Or, I take cod liver oil with a meal now and then as a substitute for omega-3. But I also make a practice of skipping both of these now and then, because too much regularity is no good; variation is better. Most fish oil capsules need to be refrigerated after opening. I recommend products that have the Star 5 rating, but am comfortable with what I find at most health food stores, drugstores, and supermarkets.

- **Melatonin:** 3 milligrams half an hour before bedtime to deepen sleep and improve antioxidants in the brain. Melatonin is a hormone secreted by the pineal gland that restores circadian rhythm and is also a powerful antioxidant to the brain. Loss of circadian rhythm and shallow sleep disturb the complexity of heart and brain dynamics and are precursors to the onset of disease. I do not take melatonin every night, but rather any time I drink coffee after noon or feel my brain is a bit too busy to fully relax. Taking a melatonin supplement every night might cause the natural release of melatonin by the pineal gland to lessen.

- **Branched-chain amino acids:** 5 grams a day with breakfast. If you're trying to gain muscle, you should take 15 grams with each meal for a week, then go off it for a week, and then alternate until you reach a healthy body composition. Women, who typically eat less meat than men but usually need to put on muscle, should take 5 to 10 grams of branched-chain amino acids three times a day, with meals. Taking this supplement will likely reduce your appetite for empty foods and increase the rate at which your body synthesizes muscle and organ mass. Men who want to add lean muscle should take the full 15 grams three times a day until they attain proper body composition. Once you've reached your desired body composition, amino acid supplements are not really necessary, though they are useful for older people who may be less active and need help to retain muscle mass.

  Branched-chain amino acid supplements are also a healthy source of protein. Exercise, combined with adequate intake of protein, promotes protein synthesis and turnover in the body, which seems to be another form of renewal that promotes health.

- **Antioxidants:** One packet with breakfast and dinner. I take a potent antioxidant supplement (Ultrathione Health Packs made by Antioxidant Pharmaceuticals Corporation) to fight inflammation. I have taken this product for 25 years and have less gray hair now than when I began, and have kept all my hair, even though it was thinning when I started (hair loss is caused by inflammation of the follicles). A key effect of inflammation is the depletion of glutathione, one of the key antioxidants present in these supplements. (I would not take any other available form of glutathione because it is digested in the stomach and may not reach the cells.) In addition to glutathione, each packet contains vitamin C, vitamin E, folic acid, and vitamin Bs 1, 2, 3, 5, 6, and 12.

As an additional countermeasure, it might be advisable to take 50 to 100 milligrams of potassium bicarbonate. This will favorably alter the sodium-potassium ratio and reduce the acid state of the body. Remember to always take a break from your supplement routine. Variation in all things—diet, exercise, and even supplements—is important.

Conclusion

A Last Word

Because this book was written by an academic, you've had to make your way through a fair amount of dense scientific information to reach this point. As a reward for your perseverance, I have boiled down the practical aspects of the New Evolution Diet to what can fit on a single page. Here are the essential principles:

- Eat fresh vegetables, fruit, nuts, meat, and fish. Stay clear of grains, legumes, potatoes, carbs, and sugar. Limit alcohol consumption.

- Skip one dinner every week.

- Exercise with intensity. Lift weights, run sprints (but don't jog or run long distances), play a sport. Your workouts should be brief and intense. Going to the gym two or three times a week, for a half hour each time, is plenty.

- Remember, the goal is to eat and exercise as humans did roughly 40,000 years ago, before the advent of agriculture or laborsaving technology. Just don't overdo it. Be glad you're here now.

- Give up the regimented approach to diet and fitness. Relax, enjoy the process, and let it happen.

Afterword

When the Human Body Needs (Extreme) Randomness

by Nassim Nicholas Taleb

Before the essayist Bryan Appleyard made the connection in his *Sunday Times* profiles, few people had been able to see the fit between my ideas on probability, empiricism, and extreme events ("Black Swans") and the diet and exercise—rather, lifestyle—views of Art De Vany. Yet they dovetail.

The story is as follows. In 2001, I published *Fooled by Randomness*, a treatise on how we overexplain matters and do not quite understand the role randomness plays in life. A few months after its publication, I received a letter from Art. He wrote these magic words to me: "I am using your book in my course on the economics of extreme events, as I despise textbooks."

They were magic because I too despise textbooks (and most textbook writers) and tend to flee what I call "serious mediocrity." My book was meant to be aggressively playful but few people noticed it consciously before Art, in spite of the sales numbers. So I knew that more mail would come from Art, but never expected it to provide the nudge that eventually changed my life.

In an e-mail, Art asked: "Do you put kurtosis into your workout?" but I did not understand why it was necessary to do so. What is kurtosis? I believed that infrequent events had a dominant role in economic life—kurtosis is the statistical name for the degree these high-impact events play into a certain distribution of outcomes—so putting kurtosis into my workout meant "Do you have moments of extreme workout?" I did not and did not realize the importance for a while.

A few facts that will follow explain that I had some of the ingredients of what I call an "ecological," nonludic way of living (avoiding what Art De Vany calls the gym equivalent of laboratory rat to living an "evolutionary" lifestyle), but didn't make an obvious connection.

1) *Lumpy Work:* I believed that only bureaucrats and other fools made a difference between work and play. The Greeks scorned what they called the banausai (artisans), the modern equivalent of salary-people, as they believed that such work led to physical (and moral) degradation. To almost all classical cultures, being involved in these routines led to muscle atrophy, and the avoidance of devotion to the life of the city led to moral decay.

Accordingly, I fought with my nails to become self-employed, with no boss to prove anything to, and I spent time doing nothing, hanging around lazily, and working with as high intensity as possible when work was necessary, for a handful of hours each week. Unpleasant tasks—like meeting with clients, talking to someone while wearing a suit and tie, talking to finance people, and listening to boring professors—needed to be dispatched as quickly as possible. Therefore, I shortened their duration and increased their intensity as far as I could. The trading life fits such a playful model as it resembles the ecology of nature and the life of a hunter: long periods of meditative inactivity, spent lounging and reading, followed by cascades of frantic and intense toil. Somehow the "doing nothing" wasn't really that, as I am certain that ideas come to those who know how to protect their intuitions from the clutter of the disease called "regular activity." Little did I know that I missed connecting the dots, stopping short of translating these ideas into a fitness regimen.

2) *Fitness:* I was then under the impression that I was fit, as I regularly rode my bicycle from the New York suburbs to my office in the Greenwich, Connecticut hills, a total of 32 miles per trip. Note that I said regularly, which, as we will see, was a mistake but I did not know it. I also ate regularly, three meals a day, which, it turns out, was an even bigger mistake. And the worst mistake: I attended a gym where I engaged in a predictably regular weight training "routine."

3) *Carbohydrate Avoidance:* Furthermore I was convinced, thanks to my father—an M.D./Ph.D. oncologist with a polymathic bent and published in many disciplines, including anthropology—of the need to avoid all carbs except for fruits. To him, an ancestral diet didn't include any source of carbohydrates other than some fruits and vegetables. But I made a mistake as I believed that we needed to eat with metronomic regularity.

My beliefs were as follows:

Inseparabilities: Just as there is this modern post-agricultural separation of work and play, you cannot separate nature from nurture, diet from work and exercise, job content from hobbies, or textbooks from reading for fun. But, under the influence of the rationalistic literature, I foolishly separated the "cardio" from the "strength" workout.

Decision Making Under Complexity: My entire body of work is based on the idea that we live in a complex system with hard-to-see causal links and an intricate web of interdependence. The human body is "opaque"; we need to rely on what had worked for a long time, hence evolution through the lengthy and merciless evolutionary test of trial-and-error, rather than any of our own theories that are deemed to be causal. Furthermore, there are nonlinearities in dose-response: A little might be beneficial, more might harm. Such nonlinearities make empiricism secondary to tradition—tradition is the result of a long series of trials and recorded in the beliefs and practices of a society that survives.

Wild Randomness: The consequence is that the randomness we observe in real life is rather more "rugged," more uneven, and more dependent on extreme outcomes than the one we study in textbooks and imagine in our mental representations. The type of randomness I call Mandelbrotian (or fractal) power laws is a different paradigm (in which extreme events play a large role) that tracks reality much better than the "bell curve" taught in schools.

Platonicity: I also believed that we make the error of rationalism, of being blinded by "what makes sense" in many fields deemed scientific, against empirical evidence—we don't like fuzziness and thus, we seek easy certainties. This leads to experts in many fields, including medicine, working with unempirical beliefs without even knowing it. So I came to think that we are suckers for "regularities" and tend to fool ourselves into believing they exist where there are none.

Evidence-Based Science & Working with the Black Box: There are methodological consequences to the opacity of the human body—the "black box." The body cannot be divorced from its environment. Mother Nature (and its logic) comes before statistics (it is a better statistician and far better biologist), but statistics come before biological theories. Furthermore, biological explanations are narrow and causal, which works poorly in a complex system, and yet we tend to be overawed by their "scientific" concreteness. As Richard Rorty wrote about a similar problem: "Sciences other than physics become 'more scientific' when they can replace functional descriptions of theoretical entities (e.g., 'gene') with structural descriptions (e.g., 'DNA molecule')."

I spent a few years reading neurobiology and papers discussing the neural correlates of decision making—how the left brain does so and so, and which neurotransmitter does what—to little avail, as simple papers in empirical psychology devoid of a single biological statement showing the result of cohort experiments turned out to be vastly more predictive. How could biologists know less than statisticians? People tend to be overawed by the scientific appearance of biological theories, against our past record—explanations change all the time. It is biologists who promoted the idea of consuming carbohydrates as a source of fuel.

To give an example of the two different approaches: People used to claim as a rationalistic theory that muscles burn more calories than fat. Now the current biological interpretation is that muscles help with insulin sensitivity, meaning that food intake does not lead to a rise of insulin in the blood. Tomorrow, someone may claim some other hormone plays a role in causing the same effect, but an empiricist would just invoke the regularity that people with more muscle mass are less flabby at an even greater caloric intake; the simple explanation is that our ancestors had more muscles than office inmates, and that's that.

The Missing 5 Minutes: Putting the Kurtosis Back

So, when in his e-mail on "kurtosis" Art asked me if I worked out in a way that was compatible with my views on extreme economics and complexity, I didn't get the point; I didn't even realize that there was an obvious divorce between my ideas on randomness and my lifestyle. Instead, I was under the rationalistic belief that exercise was exercise, and that a good life needed regular exercise; never once did I think—I never thought of looking at evidence-based papers—how exercise improved all these nice laboratory metrics but has never been proven to make people live longer. I was making two very severe mistakes: eating and working out steadily, which was not what Mother Nature built us to do. I never looked at the empirical evidence.

Nor had I realized it right away. For I was punished when, hit with boredom in Greenwich, I moved the office back to New York City and decided to replace my bicycling with gym attendance. I attended the gym as much as I used to ride my bike yet saw myself swelling, catching close to 25 pounds of adipose tissue in 3 years. Then I realized the following: I didn't understand the application of my own ideas on complexity and randomness. The reason that I was fit didn't come from the hours of bicycling I did every week, but from the two or three grueling hills on my ride that pushed my heartbeat to about 210 beats per minute—only

5 minutes of severe straining workout every ride, but these 5-minute periods were all that mattered. When I realized that fact, everything came to me in a flash, with the usual shame at not having properly connected the dots. I needed to "put kurtosis into my workout." I started reading some of Art's materials and looking for what insights evidence-based papers could offer us, all the while showing Art the pictures of the stronger and leaner body. Three years later, the improvement hasn't stopped.

There is a need for environmental randomness: So I failed in applying my ideas on Platonicity and had a representation of human life that relied on regularities and certainties. The human body is a machine fit for a certain set of random outcomes, and so it needs randomness, not predictability. We have been built under a set number of variations coming from the environment, a variety of stressors, and now we are Platonifying ourselves by depriving our lives of these variations.

So I will discuss the following two points in sequence: a) the need to put randomness into our life; b) the need to put kurtosis into such randomness.

Matching the Right Randomness to Life

A gym is to physical exercise what a chat room is to social life.

Here are the main sources of variations experienced by humans in an ancestral environment that I can think of:

- **Thermal fluctuations:** Cold, heat; add to that dryness, wetness, and high variations in humidity.

- **Energy expenditure:** Some days and seasons require more work than others, with periods of overexertion followed by long stretches of rest. Art showed, backed by research, that regular jogging and marathon running degrades your health, while sprinting and interval training improves it. Walking is not "for exercise"; like sleep, it has to be a mysteriously effective activity that is necessary for humans to operate, and it needs to be done slowly. We need to look at it the way we look at yoga and meditation.

* **Energy intake:** Bouts of hunger, fasting, followed by feast. Add to that episodes of thirst. I never have difficulty making people understand that a training workout that stresses the body is beneficial to them; the difficulty I've had is in making them understand that we must apply the same logic to hunger and thirst. Hunger had to provide some benefits. We often hear the recommendations, based on some rationalistic interpretation of the human body: Eat three meals a day, drink eight glasses of water, don't overdo it, yet evidence confirms the evolutionary argument and shows that intermittent fasting strengthens the human body by boosting the immune system, improving brain functions, and increasing insulin sensitivity (or something like insulin we don't know about as yet).

* **Sleep duration:** Our sleep periods had to experience some occasional variations.

* **Negative correlations amplifying energy deficits:** There has to be a negative correlation between energy intake and energy expenditure. We work hard in response to hunger; there is no natural, ecological reason to work hard if we are well fed—what's the point?—yet the prevailing wisdom doesn't seem to be aware of this elementary evolutionary logic. A predator mammal does not eat breakfast to hunt; it hunts in response to the need to get breakfast. However, I hear all these rationalistic statements (devoid of any evidence) about the need to eat a big breakfast before starting the day. To see how such nonsense is widespread, consider the following: In a *New York Times* science article, the journalist Tara

Parker-Hope answers a reader's question: "At what point before exercise should we be eating?" She writes: "I like it to be an hour before exercise. We're just talking about a fist-sized amount of food. That gives the body enough food to be available as an energy source but not so much that you'll have an upset stomach."

In such a representation, no doubt inspired by thermodynamics, you imagine your body like a car that you need to fill up with fuel before driving to your country house. (Incidentally, this can provide an illustration of the difference between linear science and complexity; complexity theory would consider the interdependence between the engine and the fuel.) Evidence-based methods show that this nutritional dogma has no supporting evidence going for it.

Art convinced me that we need to train our body to go hungry on occasion (or, at least, deprive it of carbs) while remaining active in order to burn fatty acids. It works by shutting down these on-demand sources of calories; he once explained that if we don't train our body to burn fat, we could die of hunger with plenty of adipose tissue around the waist. And research shows that people on a ketogenic (low-carb) diet eventually operate, after the detox period, as effectively as those on a high-pasta and orange juice diet. In short, the human body is a complex information machine, not an engine. Exercise conveys information, and genes up-regulate and down-regulate in response to stimuli—taking the information machine outside its normal, pre-agricultural habitat leads to the disruption of its equilibrium (or its various states of dynamic equilibria).

My De Vany Exercise

Fractality: There are some stressors our ancestors encountered once a decade, others once a year, others once a week, and others once a day. Hence a workout and diet regimen needs to match what follows.

1) No Moderate Exercise Sessions: Either too little, or too much, or way beyond what I plan to do, and with no set schedule. Never have a clear plan of how long to stay at the gym, as it's a matter of bandwidth. The range of fatigue from regular exercise does not reach all areas of the body, and so I now spend between 5 minutes and (very rarely) up to 2 hours at the gym, working out harder as I get more tired. Sometimes I go several weeks without any exercise, but my total time at the gym each month averages less than it did before the ecological regimen, and I have no routine: I don't count sets, and I have developed a preference for free weights/pullups/dips/pushups. Sometimes I just do pushups and avoid the "moderate" number 60: either 10 or 350, then nothing for a long time.

2) No Yoga—Just Long, Very Long, Walks: I am a flâneur and a thinker by profession, so my only regular activity in life is long walks, which I tend to take every day. I try to take aimless walks of between 1 and 2 hours a day, up to 5 hours daily when I travel. I also walk on uneven surfaces, which seems to stretch my back, and so I walk on rocks whenever I can. I believe that gym rats and cyclists don't do negative exercises that are necessary for spinal health. Our ancestors did not do yoga and stretching; they simply walked as an expression of being.

3) Occasional Sprints: As Art showed, sprinting is fun, playful, and short. You know it will be over quickly and are too engaged in it to look at a clock, as gym rats do, to see when it should be over.

4) No Purely Aerobic Exercise: The separation is foolish and not empirical. Avoid listening to "trainers."

5) Food Intake: No carbs that do not have a Biblical Hebrew or Doric Greek name (i.e., did not exist in the ancient Mediterranean): No oranges (only citrus), no bananas, no mangoes, or anything of that nature. Apples and grapes were acidic in taste, bittersweet. Like Art, I eat nothing out of the box. No sugar, bread, or pasta. Avoid artificial sweeteners. Rationalistic fools may tell you that it lowers the calories, but they are trapped in non-complex, non-information-theoretic thermodynamics—you don't know what sensors are activated by the taste of sweetness, what is up-regulated, or what happens to your mechanism of equilibrium-seeking. Arguments based on classical thermodynamics used by idiotic nutritionists do not take feedback loops into account. We have enough evidence of people gaining weight (and perhaps messing up their brain) with the regular use of these sweeteners.

Also I tend to eat very, very large meals on occasion, like Sunday feasts, leaving me feeling satisfied for days.

6) Starvation: Work out while starving.

So good luck with the regimen. I've been on it for close to 3 years and my intellectual production keeps getting greater.

Notes

* For all documents in Notes and Further Readings without page numbers provided, visit the author's Web site at www.arthurdevany.com.

Introduction

1. The evidence of genetic lineages is in Spencer Wells, *Deep Ancestry, Inside the Genographic Project* (Washington, DC: National Geographic, 2007). Wells writes, "As much as 89% of the European gene pool is attributed to the first hunter-gatherers whose descendants survived the last glacial maximum" (p. 51). The slight changes in the human genotype that have been discovered are evidence of continuing, but modest, evolution of humans.

Striking evidence of the similarity of modern European genes to those of our Cro-Magnon ancestors is provided by the DNA sequencing of a 28,000-year-old Cro-Magnon, reported in David Caramelli et al., "A 28,000 Years Old Cro-Magnon mtDNA Sequence Differs from All Potentially Contaminating Modern Sequences," *PLoS ONE* 3, no. 7 (2008). Their conclusion? "Therefore, at this stage it is safe to conclude that at least one Cro-Magnoid mtDNA sequence, for which contamination can be ruled out with a high degree of confidence, falls well within the range of modern human variation."

Humans continue to evolve. In a November 13, 2009, interview at Livescience, Professor Steven Hawks notes that the human brain continues to evolve and has shrunk about 10 percent in the past 5,000 years.

The selection pressure of the transition from hunting and gathering to agriculture has caused the evolution of the ability to digest lactose (the sugar in milk) and starch in some populations and resistance to malaria in others. Other genetic changes appear to alter smell and detoxify plant poisons, reflecting a shift of diet from wild foods to domesticated plants and animals. See Jonathon Pritchard et al., in *PLoS Biology* (March 2006), as summarized in the *New York Times* Science section, March 7, 2006. For evidence that the life of hunting and gathering demanded great strength and the ability to move quickly, see Daniel G. MacArthur and Kathryn N. North, "ACTN3: A Genetic Influence on Muscle Function and Athletic Performance, Exercise and Sports," *Exercise and Sport Sciences Review* 35, no. 1 (2007): 30–4. The authors discuss the evolution of a deficiency in more than a billion humans worldwide in the α–actinin-3 protein in fast-muscle fibers, which is associated with elite athletic performance in strength and sprinting speed.

Katharine Milton, in "Back to Basics: Why Foods of Wild Primates Have Relevance for Modern Human Health," *Nutrition* 16, no. 7–8 (2000), states, "To date, we know of few adaptations to diet in the human species that differentiate us from our closest living relatives, the great apes. Those identified are largely (although not exclusively) regulatory mutations such as lactase synthesis in adulthood, and unique selective pressures favoring such diet-associated mutations seem fairly well understood."

2. Westernized Australian aboriginals develop all the contemporary health problems, such as diabetes, obesity, and coronary heart disease. Kerin O'Dea, "Traditional Diet and Food Preferences of Australian Aboriginal Hunter-Gatherers," *Philosophical Transactions: Biological Sciences* 334, no. 1279 (1991): 233–41. O'Dea did a reverse experiment in which aboriginals temporarily returned to the bush for 7 weeks. There was "significant weight loss, and striking improvement in all of the abnormalities of diabetes together with a reduction in the major risk factors for coronary heart disease."

3. Michael Gurven and Hillard Kaplan, in "Longevity Among Hunter-
Gatherers: A Cross-Cultural Examination," *Population and Development Review* 33, no. 2 (2007): 321–65, show that the rate of life
expectancy at ages from 1 to 80 is lower among hunter-gatherers
than that in 18th-century Sweden, but the curve declines less steeply
among hunter-gatherers beginning at the age of 25. The modal age at
death—roughly, the most frequent age of death—is slightly higher
among hunter-gatherers than those in 18th-century Sweden. The
modal age at death is close to 80 among hunter-gatherers who survive infancy, which is not far below that in the United States in 2002,
which is 85. The mortality hazard ratio for hunter-gatherers and
those in the United States is high at early ages and falls to a value
close to one, indicating equal hazard of death in both populations, by
the age of 45.

Hunter-gatherers are 20 percent stronger than age- and weight-matched
Westerners and approximately 50 percent more fit aerobically. The
skeletal remains of late Paleolithic humans are comparable to those
of Olympic athletes. Hunter-gatherers have a high proportion of muscle relative to fat mass. See S. Boyd Eaton and Stanley B. Eaton III,
"An Evolutionary Perspective on Human Physical Activity: Implica-
tions for Health," *Comparative Biochemistry and Physiology* 136, no. 1
(2003): 153–9. Hunter-gatherers rarely develop chronic degenerative
diseases such as rising blood pressure, increased adiposity, deficient
lean body mass, elevated cholesterol, atherosclerosis, or insulin resistance; see Staffan Lindeberg et al., "Evolutionary Health Promotion,"
Preventive Medicine 34, no. 2 (2002): 119–23.

4. J. C. McPhee and R. J White, in "Physiology, Medicine, Long-Duration
Space Flight and the NSBRI," *Acta Astronautica* 53 (2003): 239–48,
describe the effects of prolonged space travel as "debilitating and
unacceptable." Eugenia Wang, in "Age-Dependent Atrophy and
Microgravity Travel: What Do They Have in Common?" *Federation
for American Societies for Experimental Biology Journal* 13 (1999):
167–74, shows that the muscle unloading that occurs in space gravity

and the increased expression of free radicals (ROS) and other markers of stress accelerate muscle atrophy in a similar manner to aging.
Couch potatoes are not exempt from this law.

5. On a varied diet and superior health, see Antonia Trichopoulou et
al., "Diet and Overall Survival in Elderly People," *British Medical
Journal* 311 (1995): 1457–60. On the varied diet of our ancestors, see
Bryan Hockett and Jonathan Haws, "Nutritional Ecology and Dia-
chronic Trends in Paleolithic Diet and Health," *Evolutionary Anthro-
pology* 12, no. 5 (2003). Also see B. N. Ames, "DNA Damage from
Micronutrient Deficiencies Is Likely to Be a Major Cause of Cancer,"
Mutation Research 475 (2001), 7–20. The importance of variety in
food intake for women and the children they bear is emphasized in
Adrianne Bendich, "Micronutrients in Women's Health and
Immune Function," *Nutrition* 17 (2001): 858–67.

Chapter 1: My Journey

1. Loren Cordain, in *The Paleo Diet: Lose Weight and Get Healthy by
Eating the Food You Were Designed to Eat* (New York: John Wiley
and Sons, 2002), thoroughly explains the eating patterns of hunter-
gatherers and shows how to adapt their foods to a modern diet.

2. Bryan Appleyard's "Evolutionary Fitness: The Diet That Really
Works," begins:

> A half-naked 71-year-old with 8% body fat and the testosterone
> levels of a boy of 18 greets me at the door of a large house over-
> looking a golf course near St George, Utah. He has the physique of
> a very fit young man and the springy, energetic demeanor of some-
> body who has cracked most of life's outstanding problems. I am
> calling on him because, ever since I heard of him, I have begun to
> look uncannily well.
>
> Two weeks earlier I had strolled into the office of the editor of
> this organ.
>
> "You look 10 years younger. Why?" he barked, as editors do.

I was 11 lb lighter than the last time he'd seen me. But he said "younger," note, not just thinner.

Chapter 2: Before You Begin: Eight Things to Measure

1. Body fat is referred to as adipose tissue. It is the largest organ in the human body, particularly in the obese. Adipose tissue is subcutaneous white fat, referred to as subcutaneous adipose tissue (SAT), or fat deep inside the viscera, referred to as visceral adipose tissue (VAT). There is brown adipose tissue, too, which is important in body weight. See Aaron M. Cypess, "Identification and Importance of Brown Adipose Tissue in Adult Humans," *New England Journal of Medicine* 360 (2009): 1–9.

Adipose tissue is an active endocrine organ that secretes many biochemicals, referred to collectively as adipokines, including leptin, adiponectin, resistin, and visfatin, as well as cytokines and chemokines, such as tumor necrosis factor-alpha, interleukin-6, and monocyte chemoattractant protein-1. See Barbara Antuna-Puente et al., "Adipokines: The Missing Link between Insulin Resistance and Obesity," *Diabetes and Metabolism* 34 (2008): 2–11; Rudolph L. Leibel et al., "Physiologic Basis for the Control of Body Fat Distribution in Humans," *Annual Review of Nutrition* 9 (1989): 417–43; Paul Farajian et al., "Obesity Indices in Relation to Cardiovascular Disease Risk Factors Among Young Adult Female Students," *British Journal of Nutrition* 99 (2008): 918–24. Further evidence of the contribution of inflammation to cardiovascular disease is described in Göran K. Hansson, "Inflammation, Atherosclerosis, and Coronary Artery Disease," *New England Journal of Medicine* 352, no. 16 (2005): 1685–95.

In "Obesity Indices," Farajian et al. conclude, "Although %BF was not associated with any of the CVD risk factors, waist circumference, waist:hip ratio and waist:height ratio were all (positively) associated with CVD risk factors."

2. Metabolic syndrome is called the "deadly quartet." It is a cluster of
the conditions of insulin resistance, impaired glucose tolerance,
abnormal blood fats, and hypertension. See Michael H. Shanik et al.,
"Insulin Resistance and Hyperinsulinemia: Is Hyperinsulinemia the
Cart or the Horse?" *Diabetes Care* 31, suppl. no. 2 (2008): S262–8.
The strongest predictor of metabolic syndrome found by Shanik et
al. is the VAT, located a few inches above the L4 vertebra of the
spine, giving the classic apple shape. Subcutaneous fat is somewhat
protective against the risks associated with large visceral fat, until it
reaches its limits of storage. Then, the fat is taken up by the VAT,
from whence it spills over into the liver, pericardium (the surround-
ing tissue of the heart), and muscle, where it damages the organs and
their function. Since a prominent waist is a sign of increased VAT,
while large hips are a sign of increased SAT, the waist-to-hip ratio is
an approximation of the VAT-to-SAT ratio, which seems to be why
the waist-to-hip ratio is a good predictor of metabolic syndrome.
Metabolic syndrome and cardiovascular and metabolic risk, and the
effect of visceral fat on the metabolism, are examined in Ellen W.
Demerath et al., "Visceral Adiposity and Its Anatomical Distribution as Predictors of the Metabolic Syndrome and Cardiometabolic
Risk Factor Levels," *American Journal of Clinical Nutrition* 88, no. 5
(2008): 1263–71.

3. Jonatan R. Ruiz et al., "Muscular Strength and Adiposity as Predictors of Adulthood Cancer Mortality in Men," *Cancer Epidemiology
Biomarkers and Prevention* 18, no. 5 (2009): 1468–76.

4. In research that has, at this writing, not yet been published, Frances
Hayes, MD, an endocrinologist at St. Vincent's University Hospital
in Dublin, Ireland, examined the effect of glucose on testosterone
levels in men at Boston's Massachusetts General Hospital. Hayes
and her colleagues examined the impact of a standard dose of glucose on testosterone levels in 74 men. The researchers administered
the oral glucose tolerance test, a screening test for diabetes that

involves having subjects drink a sugary solution (75 grams of pure glucose) and then measuring their blood sugar levels. The glucose solution decreased blood levels of testosterone by as much as 25 percent, regardless of whether the men had diabetes, pre-diabetes, or normal glucose tolerance.

The inverse relationship of insulin resistance to testosterone is developed in Michael Zitzmann, "Testosterone Deficiency, Insulin Resistance and the Metabolic Syndrome," *Nature Reviews Endocrinology* 5 (2009): 673–81.

5. John Danesh et al., "C-Reactive Protein and Other Circulating Markers of Inflammation in the Prediction of Coronary Heart Disease," *New England Journal of Medicine* 350, no. 14 (2004): 1387–97. The death of fat cells and the effect on the immune system is discussed in Saverio Cinti et al., "Adipocyte Death Defines Macrophage Localization and Function in Adipose Tissue of Obese Mice and Humans," *Journal of Lipid Research* 46, no. 11 (2005): 2347–55. Cell death increases thirtyfold in obese mice and dramatically in humans. Cell size is more important than the number of cells, meaning that the real problem begins when fat cells are so large that they become stressed.

6. Wolfram Alpha is the Google of scientific computation, using Mathematica as its engine and access to data as the raw material for its computations.

Chapter 3: The New Evolution Diet

1. Dr. Robert H. Lustig is the key researcher in this area, relating the brain and obesity in children. See Lustig, "How Our Western Environment Starves Kids' Brains," *Pediatric Annals* 35, no. 12 (2006): 905–7. He extends this analysis to show that obesity is a consequence of Western foods in his "Childhood Obesity: Behavioral Aberration or Biochemical Drive? Reinterpreting the First Law of Thermodynamics," *Nature Clinical Practice Endocrinology and Metabolism* 2, no. 8 (2006): 447–58. The tie to fast food is established

in Elvira Isganaitis and Robert H. Lustig, "Fast Food, Central Nervous System Insulin Resistance, and Obesity," *Arteriosclerosis, Thrombosis, and Vascular Biology* 25 (2005): 2451–62.

Other key researchers are Achim Peters and the scientists associated with his Selfish Brain Clinical Research Group. They are proponents of the selfish brain theory, as am I, which proposes that insulin resistance and the unwillingness to move and the drive to eat are related to the brain's attempts to preserve its glucose supply. See Peters et al., "The Selfish Brain: Competition for Energy Resources," *Neuroscience and Biobehavioral Reviews* 28, no. 2 (2004): 143–80; and the magisterial article by Peters et al., "Causes of Obesity: Looking Beyond the Hypothalamus," *Progress in Neurobiology* 81 (2007): 61–88.

See also Horst L. Fehm, Werner Kern, and Achim Peters, "The Selfish Brain: Competition for Energy Resources," *Progress in Brain Research* 153 (2006): 129–40, in which the authors note disorders in the "energy on request" process in the regulation of brain glucose and body weight. They point to the need to maintain the brain's glucose supply as central to its energy state, a factor that I refer to in my own personal history of combating my family's diabetes.

The role of the brain in life extension is discussed in Mark P. Mattson, "Brain Evolution and Lifespan Regulation: Conservation of Signal Transduction Pathways That Regulate Energy Metabolism," *Mechanisms of Ageing and Development* 123 (2002): 947–53.

It is well known that insulin can induce such a low state of brain glucose that a coma and death may occur. I lived through many brain emergencies with my wife and child. A brain lacking glucose can begin to die in just 5 seconds. The importance of the flow of energy to the brain is stressed in Fehm, Kern, and Peters, "The Selfish Brain," in which they point out that "the various organs of the body must compete for the allocation of a limited number of energy resources."

Fuels compete for utilization inside the body, and insulin resistance is a strategy the brain uses to protect its supply of glucose. A discussion of this competition and of the importance of insulin resistance is found in Ping Wang and Edwin C. M. Mariman, "Insulin Resistance in an Energy-Centered Perspective," *Physiology and Behavior* 94 (2008): 198–205.

For more research on brain function and nutrition, see Fernando Gómez-Pinilla, "Brain Foods: The Effects of Nutrients on Brain Function," *Nature Reviews Neuroscience* 9 (2008): 568–78; and Werner Kern, Jan Born, and Horst L. Fehm, "Role of Insulin in Alzheimer's Disease: Approaches Emerging from Basic Animal Research and Neurocognitive Studies in Humans," *Drug Development Research* 56, no. 3 (2002): 511–25. Does carbohydrate help or impede brain function? Chronic carbohydrate intake impedes it, though acute intake may help. See E. L. Gibson, "Carbohydrates and Mental Function: Feeding or Impeding the Brain?" *Nutrition Bulletin* 32, no. S1 (2007): 71–83.

2. Eric C. Westman et al., in "Low-Carbohydrate Nutrition and Metabolism," *American Journal of Clinical Nutrition* 86, no. 2 (2007): 276–84, argue that new nutritional strategies are needed to combat the growing menace of diabetes. They involve carbohydrate restriction as a means of shifting metabolism from glucose to fatty acids and ketones, precisely the strategy I'd developed for my family years ago. For more on carbohydrate restriction as the forgotten treatment for diabetes, see Eric C. Westman and Mary C. Vernon, "Has Carbohydrate-Restriction Been Forgotten as a Treatment for Diabetes Mellitus? A Perspective on the ACCORD Study Design," *Nutrition and Metabolism* 5, no. 10 (2008): 1–2.

3. The study by Laura A. Felicetti, Charles T. Robbins, and Lisa A. Shipley, "Dietary Protein Content Alters Energy Expenditure and Composition of the Mass Gain in Grizzly Bears (*Ursus arctos horribilis*)," *Physiological and Biochemical Zoology* 76, no. 2 (2003): 256–61, shows that bears feeding on a low-protein diet eat to fulfill their amino acid requirements and gain weight relative to bears fed a complete complement of amino acids. This same preference is shown in humans. See also B. Douglas White, Marty H. Porter, and

Roy J. Martin, "Protein Selection, Food Intake, and Body Composition in Response to the Amount of Dietary Protein," *Physiology and
Behavior* 69 (2000): 383–9.

High-protein (as opposed to high-carbohydrate) diets have a metabolic advantage. Eugene J. Fine and Richard D. Feinman,
"Thermodynamics and Metabolic Advantage of Weight Loss
Diets," *Metabolic Syndrome and Related Disorders* 1, no. 3 (2003):
1–11, show that weight loss on a high-protein diet of equal calories
to a high-carbohydrate diet without weight loss does not violate
the laws of thermodynamics. Equal calories, different results.

On the oft-repeated warnings regarding the possible hazards of a high-
protein diet, see Anssi H. Manninen, "High-Protein Weight Loss
Diets and Purported Adverse Effects: Where Is the Evidence?" *Journal of the International Society of Sports Nutrition* 1, no. 1 (2004):
45–51, which shows there is no evidence behind the warning.

Interlude: Why Our Ancestors Were Not Vegetarians

1. Michael Crawford and David Marsh, *Nutrition and Evolution* (New
Canaan, Connecticut: Keats Publishing, 1995).

The Rift Valley, the ancestral home of humans, is filled with lakes
thought to have been an important source of nutrition for the for-
mation of the human brain. See C. Leigh Broadhurst, Stephen C.
Cunnane, and Michael A. Crawford, "Rift Valley Lake Fish and
Shellfish Provided Brain-Specific Nutrition for Early Homo, *British
Journal of Nutrition* 79 (1998): 3–21.

See also Nuno Bicho and Jonathan Haws, "At the Land's End: Marine
Resources and the Importance of Fluctuations in the Coastline in
the Prehistoric Hunter-Gatherer Economy of Portugal," *Quaternary
Science Review* 27, no. 23–24 (2008): 2166–75.

Hunting is the occupation that made humans, according to Kim Hill,
"Hunting and Human Evolution," *Journal of Human Evolution* 11
(1982): 521–44. A male Aché hunter consumes almost 4 pounds of
meat per day.

Chapter 4: How to Not Eat

1. Arthur De Vany, "Why We Get Fat" (1998). I conclude in my complex modeling of the Paleolithic energy landscape:

The statistical models and simulations demonstrate the demanding energy management problem posed by the human adaptation. The solution is quite clear: Eating to restore energy reserves is a fatal strategy—set point humans are dead. In their place are humans who possess the ability to eat well in excess of energy expenditures, and to do it on an extended basis. Such was a necessary adaptation to uncertain energy expenditure and intake, which likely were distributed in a manner that spelled intermittent long spells of low intake and high expenditure. This is the prominent feature of the power law or Paretian distribution of energy expenditure and encounter rates with game. Enduring these spells required the ability to store energy in substantial amounts. More importantly, it requires an uncoupling of appetite from energy expenditure. This means that in relatively food-replete conditions and sedentary activity levels, humans must have the appetite to consume foods well in excess of energy expenditure. Given the intermittent, rare, but sometimes extreme episodes of large energy drains, an appetite mechanism that limited food intake during times of energy surplus would not be sufficient to sustain the individual during these periods of large energy deficit.

My calculations show that "energy balance is something that would be achieved over relatively long time intervals for a foraging Paleolithic human. They would have been in energy deficit as much as one third of the time and would experience some rather painfully long periods of hunger stress. But, given their intake and expenditure strategies, few would starve to death unless there were substantial shifts in the plant and prey distributions."

In Kevin R. Rarick et al., "Energy Flux, More So Than Energy Balance, Protein Intake, or Fitness Level, Influences Insulin-Like Growth Factor-I System Responses During 7 Days of Increased Physical

Activity," *Journal of Applied Physiology* 103, no. 5 (2007): 1613–21, it is shown that energy flux, rather than energy balance, influences the growth pathway.

The other primary determinant of mortality and fertility that is emphasized in the literature is micronutrient deficiencies that might result from the lack of diversity in the diet. See Elisabetta Di Cintio et al., "Dietary Factors and Risk of Spontaneous Abortion," *European Journal of Obstetrics and Gynecology and Reproductive Biology* 95 (2001): 132–6. The role of nutrition in death in the Paleolithic is developed in Lyle W. Konigsberg and Susan R. Frankenberg, "Deconstructing Death in Paleodemography," *American Journal of Physical Anthropology* 117 (2002): 297–309.

Related literature on nutritional ecology are João Zilhão, "Neanderthal/Modern Human Interaction in Europe," in "Questioning the Answers: Resolving Fundamental Problems of the Early Upper Paleolithic," ed. Paul T. Thacker and Maureen A. Hays, *British Archaeological Reports International Series* 1005 (2001): 13–9; Mark F. Teaford and Peter S. Ungar, "Diet and the Evolution of the Earliest Human Ancestors," *Proceedings of the National Academy of Sciences* 97, no. 13 (2000): 506–11; and William A. Stini, "Body Composition and Nutrient Reserves in Evolutionary Perspective," *World Review of Nutrition and Diet* 37 (1981): 55–83.

The fugitive nature of game and the importance of meat is discussed in John D. Speth, "Early Hominid Hunting and Scavenging: The Role of Meat as an Energy Source," *Journal of Human Evolution* 18 (1989): 329–43.

2. A good deal of aging research has focused on the insulin-IGF-1 pathway, implicating insulin as a key component of the aging pathways. Since insulin is deeply involved in glucose metabolism and storage, this suggests that glucose may be an important signal of the aging mechanisms. The insulin-IGF-1 pathway is ancient and exists in most organisms. When nutrients are abundant, the insulin-IGF signaling (IIS) pathway promotes growth and energy

storage but shortens life span, see Meng C. Wang, Dirk Bohmann, and Heinrich Jasper, "JNK Extends Life Span and Limits Growth by Antagonizing Cellular and Organism-Wide Responses to Insulin Signaling," *Cell* 121, no. 1 (2005): 115–25.

On how ancient this pathway is, see Michelangela Barbieri et al., "Insulin/IGF-I-Signaling Pathway: An Evolutionarily Conserved Mechanism of Longevity from Yeast to Humans," *American Journal of Physiology–Endocrinology and Metabolism* 285 (2003): E1064–71.

Dramatic new results that directly implicate glucose in longevity can be found in Seung-Jae Lee, Coleen T. Murphy, and Cynthia Kenyon, "Glucose Shortens the Life Span of *C. elegans* by Downregulating DAF-16/FOXO Activity and Aquaporin Gene Expression," *Cell Metabolism* 10, no. 5 (2009): 379–91. This important study caused the researchers to drop sugars and simple starches from their diets immediately following their discovery and is summarized in "Certain Proteins Extend Life Span in Worms by 30 Percent," ScienceDaily, www.sciencedaily.com/releases/2010/06/100616133319.htm.

Following Lee, Murphy, and Kenyon's worm results, University of Alabama at Birmingham researchers found that in humans "restricting consumption of glucose, the most common dietary sugar, can extend the life of healthy human-lung cells and speed the death of precancerous human-lung cells, reducing cancer's spread and growth rate." "Calorie Intake Linked to Cell Lifespan, Cancer Development," ScienceDaily, www.sciencedaily.com/releases/2009/12/091217183053.htm.

Stress resistance through calorie restriction is discussed in Byung P. Yu and Hae Young Chung, "Stress Resistance by Caloric Restriction for Longevity," *Annals of the New York Academy of Sciences* 928 (2001): 39–47. Richard Weindruch et al., "Gene Expression Profiling of Aging Using DNA Microarrays," *Mechanisms of Ageing and Development* 123 (2002): 177–93, shows significant alteration of aging-related gene expression under calorie restriction.

The New Evolution Diet is relatively low in calories and assures a balanced amino acid profile. According to research, this combination may reduce aging. See "Balancing Protein Intake, Not Cutting Calories, May Be Key to Long Life," ScienceDaily, December 6, 2009, www.sciencedaily.com/releases/2009/12/091202131622.htm.

3. Brain nutrition is compromised in anorexia, and some parts of the brain decline in mass; see Angela Wagnerad et al., "Normal Brain Tissue Volumes after Long-Term Recovery in Anorexia and Bulimia Nervosa," *Biological Psychiatry* 59, no. 3 (2006): 291–3. Gray matter is decreased in the anterior cingulate of anorexics; see Mark Mühlau et al., "Gray Matter Decrease of the Anterior Cingulate Cortex in Anorexia Nervosa," *American Journal of Psychiatry* 164 (2007): 1850–7.

4. Intermittent-fasting experiments in animals and humans are reviewed in Krista A. Varady and Marc K. Hellerstein, "Alternate-Day Fasting and Chronic Disease Prevention: A Review of Human and Animal Trials," *American Journal of Clinical Nutrition* 86 (2007): 77–88; Marcela Sene-Fiorese et al., "Efficiency of Intermittent Exercise on Adiposity and Fatty Liver in Rats Fed with High-Fat Diet," *Obesity* 16, no. 10 (2008): 2217–22; Nils Halberg et al., "Effect of Intermittent Fasting and Refeeding on Insulin Action in Healthy Men," *Journal of Applied Physiology* 99 (2005): 2128–36; and Matthew D. W. Piper and Andrzej Bartke, "Diet and Aging," *Cell Metabolism* 8, no. 2 (2008): 99–104.

5. Female mutant mice lacking the insulin-IGF receptor live 33 percent longer than others. See Marc Tatar, Andrzej Bartke, and Adam Antebi, "The Endocrine Regulation of Aging by Insulin-Like Signals," *Science* 299, no. 5611 (2003): 1346–51, which is taken as evidence of this pathway's role in aging and longevity.

6. Our little *C. elegans* worm experiences an increased life span under glucose restriction; see Tim J. Schulz et al., "Glucose Restriction Extends *Caenorhabditis elegans* Life Span by Inducing Mitochondrial Respiration and Increasing Oxidative Stress," *Cell Metabolism* 6 (2007): 280–93.

7. Further support for glucose restriction is in the remarkable finding that switching metabolism to glycolysis, of the sort stimulated by intense exercise, may induce the longevity effects of chronic caloric restriction in yeast and other organisms that share the same pathways activated by caloric restriction (humans share those pathways). See Min Wei et al., "Tor1/Sch9-Regulated Carbon Source Substitution Is as Effective as Calorie Restriction in Life Span Extension," *PLoS Genetics* 5, no. 5 (2009).

8. On brains and obesity, see Cyrus A. Raji et al., "Brain Structure and Obesity," *Human Brain Mapping* 31, no. 3 (2009): 353–64. Michael A. Ward et al., in "The Effect of Body Mass Index on Global Brain Volume in Middle-Aged Adults: A Cross Sectional Study," *BioMed-Central Neurology* 5, no. 23 (2005), found that elevated BMI is associated with lesser brain volume in middle-age adults (mean age = 54 years) even after adjusting for age. Nicola Pannacciulli et al., in "Brain Abnormalities in Human Obesity: A Voxel-Based Morphometric Study," *Neuroimage* 31 (2006): 1419–25, find that in comparison with the group of lean subjects, the group of obese individuals had significantly lower gray matter density in the postcentral gyrus, frontal operculum, putamen, and middle frontal gyrus after adjustment for sex, age, handedness, global tissue density, and multiple comparisons. BMI was negatively associated with gray matter density of the left post-central gyrus in obese subjects but not lean ones. William Jagust et al., in "Central Obesity and the Aging Brain," *Archives of Neurology* 62, no. 10 (2005): 1545–8, show that brain mass is reduced as the waist-to-hip ratio increases.

9. More on glucose restriction is found in Antoine E. Roux et al., "Pro-Aging Effects of Glucose Signaling through a G Protein-Coupled Glucose Receptor in Fission Yeast," *PLoS Genetics* 5, no. 3 (2009): 1–17. Stress resistance through calorie restriction is discussed in Yu and Chung, "Stress Resistance by Caloric Restriction."

Even a brief binge on glucose alters gene expression unfavorably. The persisting alteration of gene expression following those holiday "I'll just do it this one time" binging episodes is described in Assam El-Osta et al., "Transient High Glucose Causes Persistent Epigenetic Changes and Altered Gene Expression during Subsequent Normo-glycemia," *Journal of Experimental Medicine* 205, no. 10 (2008): 2409–17. This is the mechanism behind the metabolic memory that I had found in my first wife's blood sugars following a big bowl of spaghetti or an episode of low blood glucose.

A simple diet for glucose restriction is the one promoted here, which is known as the Paleolithic, hunter-gatherer diet. See Lynda A. Frassetto et al., "Metabolic and Physiologic Improvements from Consuming a Paleolithic, Hunter-Gatherer Type Diet," *European Journal of Clinical Nutrition* 63 (2009): 947–55.

10. Intermittent fasting confers benefits that do not depend on restricting calories. R. Michael Anson and his co-authors report that when " . . . mice are maintained on an intermittent fasting (alternate-day fasting) dietary-restriction regimen their overall food intake is not decreased and their body weight is maintained. Nevertheless, intermittent fasting resulted in beneficial effects that met or exceeded those of caloric restriction including reduced serum glucose and insulin levels and increased resistance of neurons in the brain to excitotoxic stress. Intermittent fasting therefore has beneficial effects on glucose regulation and neuronal resistance to injury in these mice that are independent of caloric intake. See Anson et al. Intermittent fasting dissociates beneficial effects of dietary restriction on glucose metabolism and neuronal resistance to injury from calorie intake. Proceedings of the *National Academy of Sciences* (2003): vol. 100 (10) 6216–20.

Chapter 5: A Month on the New Evolution Diet

1. See Robert Wolfe, "The Underappreciated Role of Muscle in Health and Disease," *American Journal of Clinical Nutrition* 84, no. 3 (2006): 1–8.

Unlike the typical male, who loses muscle mass with age, I have

retained the muscle mass of my youth and have weighed within 5
pounds of what I weighed at age 17, while retaining or increasing
the muscle mass I had at that age. The typical male loses 2 kilograms of muscle mass every decade starting in his twenties. The
causes are inadequate stimulus to the muscle and its activating
neurons, inadequate protein intake, and inflammation (which kills
fast-twitch muscle fiber).

On the muscle mass of aged males, see Vernon R. Young, "Amino
Acids and Proteins in Relation to the Nutrition of Elderly People,"
Age and Ageing 19, suppl. no. 1 (1990): S10–24. Young puts the
muscle mass of a "normal" male my age at 13 kilograms—which is
pitiful. Mine is closer to 30 kilograms.

Eugenia Wang, "Age-Dependent Atrophy and Microgravity Travel:
What Do They Have in Common?" *FASEB Journal* 13 (1999):
S167–74, compares the loss of muscle due to aging with the low-
gravity loading of muscle and skeleton that happens in space
flight. On inadequate protein intake in the aged, see Anna E.
Thalaker-Mercer et al., "Inadequate Protein Intake Affects Skel-
etal Muscle Transcript Profiles in Older Humans," *Physiological
Genomics* 85, no. 5 (2007): 1344–52.

2. Feinman and Fine, "Thermodynamics and Metabolic Advantage of
Weight Loss Diets," *Metabolic Syndrome and Related Disorders*
2005): vol. 1 (3) 1–11. They say: In summary, the need to meet the
obligate demand for glucose means that a nominally eucaloric low
carbohydrate diet can lead to increased gluconeogenesis from protein. Increased gluconeogenesis will, in turn, lead to protein turnover. Together, these processes will lead to weight loss. Leucine and
alanine are primary substrates for gluconeogenesis.

3. The difficulty people have in following a diet is more than psychological; it is physiological. Physiology trumps psychology. The
physiological reason for this is that a brain lacking glucose
because of the "deadly duo" of high insulin and high cortisol has
no willpower; it thinks it is starving and does not have the glucose required to exercise willpower. See Matthew T. Gailliot and

Roy F. Baumeister, "The Physiology of Willpower: Linking Blood
Glucose to Self-Control," *Personality and Social Psychology Review*
11 (2007): 303–27; and Huiyuan Zheng and Hans-Rudi Berthoud,
"Neural Systems Controlling the Drive to Eat: Mind versus
Metabolism," *Physiology* 23, no. 2 (2008): 75–83.

4. When insulin secretion is decreased through weight loss, food preferences are altered in favor of foods other than carbohydrates, and
appetite diminishes. P. A. Velasquez-Mieyer et al., "Suppression of
Insulin Secretion Is Associated with Weight Loss and Altered Macronutrient Intake and Preference in a Subset of Obese Adults,"
International Journal of Obesity and Related Metabolic Disorders 27,
no. 3 (2003): 219–26.

While fatty liver is usually associated with alcoholics, it is now
common among the obese and even in children. See Jeffrey D.
Browning et al., "A Low-Carbohydrate Diet Rapidly and Dramatically Reduces Intrahepatic Triglyceride Content," *Hepatology* 44,
no. 2 (2006): 487–8. This study shows the dramatic effect of a
low-carbohydrate diet and moderate exercise on the fatty acid
content of the liver. When triglycerides were mobilized from the
liver, glucose production in the liver increased, meaning the
brain's glucose was being supplied by the liver rather than from
the carbohydrates that were eaten.

The connection between stress hormones and food preference
and intake is reviewed in Mary F. Dallman et al., "Minireview:
Glucocorticoids—Food Intake, Abdominal Obesity, and Wealthy
Nations in 2004," *Endocrinology* 145, no. 6 (2004): 2633–8. Individuals with high stress hormone levels and high insulin chose to
eat more calories from sweet and fat foods. Insulin and cortisol
are called the "deadly duo" for their profound effect on consumption of sweet, high-fat foods.

A science-drenched but readable discussion of stress is Robert M.
Sapolsky's *Why Zebras Don't Get Ulcers,* 3rd ed. (New York: Henry
Holt and Company, 2004). How stress, inflammation, and metabo-
lism are intertwined is covered in Kathryn E. Wellen and Gökhan

S. Hotamisligil, "Inflammation, Stress, and Diabetes," *Journal of Clinical Investigation* 115, no. 5 (2005): 1111–9; and Dallman et al., "Minireview: Glucocorticoids."

The failure of feedback loops to control stress is shown in Mary F. Dallman et al., "Stress, Feedback and Facilitation in the Hypothalamo-Pituitary-Adrenal Axis," *Journal of Neuroendocrinology* 4, no. 5 (1992): 517–26.

On exercise being good for the brain, see Carl W. Cotman and Nicole C. Berchtold, "Exercise: A Behavioral Intervention to Enhance Brain Health and Plasticity," *Trends in Neurosciences* 25 (2002): 295–301. I do have a problem with them calling exercise an "intervention," but I always feel better after exercising, and it is because of the way exercise or play releases brain neurotrophic factor (a kind of growth hormone for neurons).

Interlude: The Worst Foods You Can Eat

1. High-carb foods that are loaded with fat, such as the french fry, raise blood glucose and the fats circulating in the bloodstream. Elevated blood glucose promotes the formation of ROS, which causes oxidative stress. If there are substantial fats associated with the carbohydrates in french fries that produce hyperglycemia, that can also contribute to oxidative stress. See George King and Mary Loeken, "Hyperglycemia-Induced Oxidative Stress in Diabetic Complications," *Histochemistry and Cell Biology* 122 (2004): 333–8; and Melvin R. Hayden and Suresh C. Tyagi, "Intimal Redox Stress: Accelerated Atherosclerosis in Metabolic Syndrome and Type 2 Diabetes Mellitus." *Cardiovascular Diabetology* 1, no. 3 (2002).

Richard Wood et al., "Effects of a Carbohydrate-Restricted Diet on Emerging Plasma Markers for Cardiovascular Disease," *Nutrition and Metabolism* 32, no. 19 (2006): 1–12. Kaye Foster-Powell, Susanna H. A. Holt, and Janette C. Brand-Miller, "International Table of Glycemic Index and Glycemic Load Values," *American Journal of Clinical Nutrition* 76, no. 1 (2002): 5–56, reports that oxidative stress and elevated coagulation from transient glycemia, following a high-glycemic-load food such as a french fry, cause "excessive postprandial glycemia [that] could decrease blood HDL-cholesterol concentrations, increase triglyceridemia, and also be directly toxic by increasing protein glycation, generating oxidative stress, and causing transient hypercoagulation and impaired endothelial function." In other words, the thickened blood resulting from elevated blood glucose could impair the blood vessels. When they go into spasm and constrict, a heart attack can result. Alan W. Barclay et al., "Glycemic Index, Glycemic Load, and Chronic Disease Risk: A Meta-analysis of Observational Studies," *American Journal of Clinical Nutrition* 87, no. 3 (2008): 627–37, is a meta-study of glycemic load and disease risk in which the authors conclude that their findings support the hypothesis that higher postprandial (after eating) glycemia is a universal mechanism for disease progression.

2. By Mary Kay Fox, MEd; Susan Pac, M.S., R.D.; Barbara Devaney, Ph.D; and Linda Jankowski, M.S., "Feeding Infants and Toddlers Study: What Foods Are Infants and Toddlers Eating?" *Journal of the American Dietetic Association* 104, (2004): S22–30.

Chapter 6: How to Exercise

1. Lewis A. Lipsitz, "Dynamics of Stability: The Physiologic Basis of Functional Health and Frailty," *Journals of Gerontology, Series A* 57A, no. 3 (2002): B115–25.

Mikko Tulppo et al., "Effects of Exercise and Passive Head-Up Tilt on Fractal and Complexity Properties of Heart Rate Dynamics," *American Journal of Physiology* 280, no. 3 (2001): H1061–7.

On weight lifting improving heart rate dynamics, see Kevin S. Heffernan et al., "Fractal Scaling Properties of Heart Rate Dynamics Following Resistance Exercise Training," *Journal of Applied Physiology* 105 (2008): 109–113. On how disease and aging reduce fractal dynamics, see Ary L. Goldberger et al., "Fractal Dynamics in Physiology: Alterations with Disease and Aging," *Proceedings of the National Academy of Sciences* 99, suppl. no. 1 (2002): 2466–72.

Bruce West, *Where Medicine Went Wrong: Rediscovering the Path to Complexity* (Singapore: World Scientific, 2006), shows the errors that result from considering the body to be a simple system, even multiple simple systems, and offers a way of replacing traditional physiology with a fractal physiology based on complexity.

2. The "runner's high" is sometimes described as a state of harmony or euphoria. This is brain chemistry. Henning Boecker et al., "The Runner's High: Opioidergic Mechanisms in the Human Brain," *Cerebral Cortex* 18 (2008): 2523–31. Pet scans revealed that sustained exercise released endogenous opioids in frontal regions of the brain. C. L. Chapman and J. M. De Castro point to this as a source of addiction to excessive sports in "Running Addiction: Measurement and Associated Psychological Characteristics," *Journal of Sports Medicine and Physical Fitness* 30 (1990): 283–90.

Weight lifting relieves depression among the elderly because it promotes a sense of self-efficacy. Nalin A. Singh, Karen M. Clements, and Maria A. Fiatarone, "A Randomized Controlled Trial of Progressive Resistance Training in Depressed Elders," *Journal of Gerontology* 57A, no. 1 (1997): M27–35.

3. Marcela Sene-Fiorese et al., "Efficiency of Intermittent Exercise on Adiposity and Fatty Liver in Rats Fed with High-Fat Diet," *Obesity* 16, no. 10 (2008): 2217–22. A. J. Schwarz et al., "Acute Effect of Brief Low- and High-Intensity Exercise on Circulating Insulin-Like Growth Factor (IGF) I, II, and IGF-Binding Protein-3 and Its Proteolysis in Young Healthy Men," *Journal of Clinical Endocrinology and Metabolism* 81 (1996): 3592–7. On exercise mimicking the effects of dietary restriction on life span, see Eric T. Poehlman et al., "Caloric Restriction Mimetics Physical Activity and Body Composition Changes," *Journals of Gerontology, Series A* 56A (2001): 45–54.

G. D. Wadley et al., "Effect of Exercise Intensity and Hypoxia on Skeletal Muscle AMPK Signaling and Substrate Metabolism in

Humans," *American Journal of Physiology—Endocrinology and Metabolism* 290 (2006): E694–702.

4. Simon Melov et al., "Resistance Exercise Reverses Aging in Human Skeletal Muscle," *PLoS ONE* 2, no. 5 (2007). The expression of 179 genes associated with aging were normalized with exercise, which is to say those that reduce aging were expressed more and those that increase aging were reduced. On exercise also altering gene expression in the brain, see Liqi Tong et al., "Effects of Exercise on Gene-Expression Profile in the Rat Hippocampus," *Neurobiology of Disease* 8, no. 6 (2001): 1046–65. On exercise altering the functional impairment of aging, see David R. Thomas, "The Critical Link Between Health-Related Quality of Life and Age-Related Changes in Physical Activity and Nutrition," *Journals of Gerontology, Series A* 56A, no. 10 (2001): M599–602.

5. We do judge people harshly for being fat, and this may be a stigma that began during evolutionary times, when obesity was rare and almost surely indicated that that person was taking more from the group than they were contributing to it. Jeffrey M. Friedman, "Modern Science versus the Stigma of Obesity," *Nature Medicine* 10, no. 6 (2004): 563–9, suggests that this anachronistic attitude may get in the way of good science.

6. Kim Hill lived and hunted with the Aché. Their physical prowess is documented in his article "Hunting and Evolution," *Journal of Human Evolution* 11 (1982): 521–44. He says this about them: "I used to train for marathons as a grad student and could run at a 6:00 per mile pace for 10 miles, but the Aché would run me into the ground following peccary tracks through dense bush for a couple of hours. I did the 100 yd in 10.2 in high school (I was a fast pass catcher on my football team), and some Aché men can sprint as fast as me."

7. The obesity gene, known as the "ob gene," is expressed in adipose tissues. The ob gene controls fat storage and is regulated by exercise, nutrition, and hormones. Donghai Zheng et al., "The Effect of

Exercise on Ob Gene Expression," *Biochemical and Biophysical Research Communications* 225 (1996): 747–50. This paper shows that a single bout of exercise decreased ob gene messenger RNA levels (mRNA) immediately, a decrease that lasted up to 3 hours after exercise. Fasting and exercise decrease the expression of the ob gene; insulin and feeding increase it.

Exercising in the fasted state promotes fat utilization. See Anthony A. Civitarese et al., "Glucose Ingestion during Exercise Blunts Exercise-Induced Gene Expression of Skeletal Muscle Fat Oxidative Genes," *American Journal of Physiology—Endocrinology and Metabolism* 289 (2005): E1023–9; and K. De Bock, "Exercise in the Fasted State Facilitates Fibre Type-Specific Intramyocellular Lipid Breakdown and Stimulates Glycogen Resynthesis in Humans," *Journal of Physiology* 564 (2005): 649–60.

8. A general discussion of the overtraining syndrome is A. Angeli et al., "The Overtraining Syndrome in Athletes: A Stress-Related Disorder," *Journal of Endocrinological Investigation* 6 (2004): 603–12. The authors summarize it thusly: "Athletes undergoing a strenuous training schedule can develop a significant decrease in performance associated with systemic symptoms or signs: the overtraining syndrome (OTS). This is a stress-related condition that consists of alteration of physiological functions and adaptation to performance, impairment of psychological processing, immunological dysfunction and biochemical abnormalities. With excessive repetition of the training stimulus the local inflammation can generate a systemic inflammatory response."

On overtraining suppressing the immune system and elevating stress to a chronic form, see M. Gleeson, G. I. Lancaster, and N. C. Bishop, "Nutritional Strategies to Minimise Exercise-Induced Immunosuppression in Athletes," *Canadian Journal of Applied Physiology* 26 (2001): S23–35; Mark Parry-Billings et al., "Plasma Amino Acid Concentration in the Overtraining Syndrome: Possible Effects on the Immune System," *Medicine and Science in Sports and Exercise*

24, no. 12 (1992): 1353–8; and D. C. Nieman et al., "Infectious Episodes in Runners before and after the Los Angeles Marathon," *Journal of Sports Medicine and Physical Fitness* 30 (1990): 316–28.

On overtraining increasing gut permeability, see Kay L. Pals et al.,
"Effect of Running Intensity on Intestinal Permeability," *Journal of
Applied Physiology* 82 (1997): 571–6.

On overtraining causing inflammation, see Lucille Lakier Smith,
"Cytokine Hypothesis of Overtraining: A Physiological Adaptation
to Excessive Stress?" *Medicine and Science in Sports and Exercise* 32
(2000): 317–31.

Interlude: Boys to Girls

1. Obese males (and females) aromatize excessive amounts of testosterone to estrogen; see M. A. Kirschner et al., "Obesity, Androgens,
   Estrogens, and Cancer Risk," *Cancer Research* 42 (1982): 3281–5.
   The inverse relationship of insulin resistance to testosterone is
   developed in Michael Zitzmann, "Testosterone Deficiency, Insulin
   Resistance and the Metabolic Syndrome," *Nature Reviews Endocrinology* 5 (2009): 673–81.

2. Read this text from Anna-Maria Andersson et al., "Secular Decline
   in Male Testosterone and Sex Hormone Binding Globulin Serum
   Levels in Danish Population Surveys," *Journal of Clinical Endocrinology and Metabolism* 92, no. 12 (2007): 4696–4706, and try not to
   weep for Sunday-football males: "Alternatively, cross-sectional data
   on the older age ranges may be biased toward containing a higher
   proportion of healthy men, compared with the younger age ranges,
   implying that unhealthy men are less likely to become old. However, yet another alternative explanation could be that a secular
   decline in testosterone levels exists, because men studied 20 yr ago
   had higher serum testosterone levels than men of the same age
   studied today."

3. On declining free testosterone as a predictor of the metabolic
   syndrome, see David E. Laaksonen et al., "Testosterone and Sex

Hormone–Binding Globulin Predict the Metabolic Syndrome and
Diabetes in Middle-Aged Men," *Diabetes Care* 27, no. 5 (2004):
1036–41.

4. On the general decline with aging of metabolism and body composition, as well as the role of testosterone in this process, see Ronenn
Roubenoff and Laura C. Rall, "Humoral Mediation of Changing
Body Composition during Aging and Chronic Inflammation,"
Nutrition Reviews 51, no. 1 (1993): 1–11; and Annewieke W. van den
Beld et al., "Measures of Bioavailable Serum Testosterone and Estra-
diol and Their Relationships with Muscle Strength, Bone Density,
and Body Composition in Elderly Men," *Journal of Clinical Nutrition*
86, no. 9 (2000): 3276–82. On the association of stress and poor
metabolism with low testosterone, see Constantine Tsigos and
George P. Chrousos, "Hypothalamic-Pituitary-Adrenal Axis, Neuro-
endocrine Factors and Stress," *Journal of Psychosomatic Research* 53
(2002): 865–71. An excellent review of the determinants of muscle
mass, including testosterone, is Michael J. Rennie et al., "Control of
the Size of the Human Muscle Mass," *Annual Reviews of Physiology*
66 (2004): 799–828.

Testosterone level is a better predictor than leptin of mortality in aged
males; see Simon et al., "Serum Testosterone But Not Leptin Predicts Mortality in Elderly Men," *Research Letters: Ageing* (2008),
published electronically. See Chapter 1, footnote 4.

5. On alcohol as a prime contributor to hypogonadism and feminization of males; see G. G. Gordon, A. L. Southern, and C. S. Lieber,
"Hypogonadism and Feminization in the Male: A Triple Effect of
Alcohol," *Alcoholism: Clinical and Experimental Research* 3 (1979):
210–2.

Chapter 7: The Metaphysics Behind the Diet

1. Nassim Taleb, *The Black Swan* (New York: Random House, 2007).
2. On exercise improving the fractal and dynamics properties of the

heartbeat, see Mikko Tulppo et al., "Effects of Exercise and Passive Head-Up Tilt on Fractal and Complexity Properties of Heart Rate Dynamics," *American Journal of Physiology* 280, no. 3 (2001): H1061–7; and Kevin S. Heffernan et al., "Fractal Scaling Properties of Heart Rate Dynamics Following Resistance Exercise Training," *Journal of Applied Physiology* 105 (2008): 109–13.

The dynamics of physiology as a model of functional health is reviewed in Lewis A. Lipsitz, "Dynamics of Stability: The Physiologic Basis of Functional Health and Frailty," *Journals of Gerontology, Series A* 57A, no. 3 (2002): B115–25. For a restatement of how the new fractal physiology alters the idea of maintaining homeostasis in favor of dynamic adaptation, see Ary L. Goldberger et al., "Fractal Dynamics in Physiology: Alterations with Disease and Aging," *Proceedings of the National Academy of Sciences* 99, suppl. no. 1 (2002): 2466–72.

Interlude: Sir Steven and Michael Phelps

1. K. De Bock et al., "Effect of Training in the Fasted State on Metabolic Responses during Exercise with Carbohydrate Intake," *Journal of Applied Physiology* 104, no. 4 (2008): 1045–55.

2. Stephen D. Phinney, "Ketogenic Diets and Physical Performance," *Nutrition and Metabolism* 1, no. 1 (2004): 2; and Stephen D. Phinney et al., "The Human Metabolic Response to Chronic Ketosis without Caloric Restriction: Preservation of Submaximal Exercise Capability with Reduced Carbohydrate Oxidation," *Metabolism* 32 (1983): 769–76.

Chapter 8: The Competition Within

1. William R. Leonard and Marcia L. Robertson, "Nutritional Requirements and Human Evolution: A Bioenergetics Model," *American Journal of Human Biology* 4, no. 2 (1992): 179–95.

2. Jeffrey S. Flier, "What's in a Name? In Search of Leptin's Physiologic Role 1," *Journal of Clinical Endocrinology and Metabolism* 83, no. 5

(1998): 1404–13. Flier states, "I have reviewed some of the reasons why a response to starvation might be retained, whereas the response to limit obesity, despite its value in a world of nutritional excess, might have been selected against by evolution, accounting for the high prevalence of obesity in the modern world."

Jameason Cameron and Éric Doucet, in "Getting to the Bottom of Feeding Behavior: Who's on Top?" *Applied Physiology* 32, no. 1 (2007): 177–81, argue that evolution has selected for a system of energy regulation that sets a lower limit on stores of energy in adipose tissues, but not an upper limit. This is what I found in my simulations of the Paleolithic energy landscape in my "Why We Get Fat."

Kathryn E. Wellen and Gökhan S. Hotamisligil, in "Inflammation, Stress, and Diabetes," *Journal of Clinical Investigation* 115, no. 5 (2005): 1111–19, hypothesize that inflammation is an adaptive response of metabolism to excess body fat and "that mechanisms such as the activation of catabolism via inflammation (and hence resistance to anabolic signals) may be an attempt to keep body weight within acceptable bounds." In other words, the immune system attacks fat as though it were a tumor.

3. Ellen W. Demerath et al., "Visceral Adiposity and Its Anatomical Distribution as Predictors of the Metabolic Syndrome and Cardiometabolic Risk Factor Levels," *American Journal of Clinical Nutrition* 88, no. 5 (2008): 1263–71. Their chilling finding, among others, is "increased metabolic risk stems from exceeding the capacity of the subcutaneous adipocytes to differentiate and accommodate excess circulating lipids, which results in ectopic deposition of lipids—that is, deposition in the liver, muscles, pericardium, and visceral compartments."

4. Aging and loss of muscle mass seem to be caused by inflammation. See A. M. Solomon and P. M. G. Bouloux, "Modifying Muscle Mass— the Endocrine Perspective," *Journal of Endocrinology* 191 (2006): 349–60. You can see images of inflamed fat caused by macrophage infiltration to mop up the debris from the death of supersize fat cells

in Saverio Cinti et al., "Adipocyte Death Defines Macrophage Localization and Function in Adipose Tissue of Obese Mice and Humans,"
Journal of Lipid Research 46, no. 11 (2005): 2347–55. I think aging is
an inflammatory disease, as spelled out in B. N. Ames, M. K. Shi-
genaga, and T. M. Hagen, "Oxidants, Antioxidants, and the Degenerative Diseases of Aging," *Proceedings of the National Academy of
Sciences* 90, no. 17 (1993): 7915–22.

5. See Demerath et al., "Visceral Adiposity"; and Harold Bays, Lawrence Mandarino, and Ralph A. DeFronzo, "Role of the Adipocyte,
Free Fatty Acids, and Ectopic Fat in Pathogenesis of Type 2 Diabetes Mellitus: Peroxismal Proliferator-Activated Receptor Agonists
Provide a Rational Therapeutic Approach," *Journal of Clinical Endocrinology and Metabolism* 89, no. 2 (2004): 463–78.

6. Skeletal muscle is called an organ because it produces and releases
cytokines, which have been named "myokines." Muscle is the largest
organ in the human body, so the concept that it releases signaling
chemicals is a new model of the effects of exercise. See Anne Marie
W. Petersen and Bente Klarlund Pedersen, "The Anti-Inflammatory
Effect of Exercise," *Journal of Applied Physiology* 98 (2005): 1154–62;
and Bente Klarlund Pedersen and Mark Febbraio, "Muscle-Derived
Interleukin-6—A Possible Link between Skeletal Muscle, Adipose Tissue, Liver, and Brain," *Brain Behavior and Immunity* 19 (2005): 371–6.

Chapter 9: Age Like Me

1. Those most likely to fall are obese and sarcopenic, meaning they
have lost muscle mass. Baumgartner, "Body Composition in
Healthy Aging," *Annals of the New York Academy of Sciences*
(2000), vol. 904: 437–48. Obese sarcopenic men are nine times
more likely to have three or more disabilities and, for women, the
risk is 12 times higher than the baseline risk. The risk of falls is
3.34 to 2.12 times higher respectively.

2. Simon Melov et al., "Resistance Exercise Reverses Aging in Human
Skeletal Muscle," *PLoS ONE* 2, no. 5 (2007); and David R. Thomas,

"The Critical Link between Health-Related Quality of Life and Age-Related Changes in Physical Activity and Nutrition," *Journals of Gerontology, Series A* 56A, no. 1 (2001): M599–602.

3. My low insulin is crucial to slowing the rate at which I am aging. Akiko Taguchi and Morris F. White, "Insulin-Like Signaling, Nutrient Homeostasis, and Life Span," *Annual Review of Physiology* 70 (2009): 191–212. Nora Klöting and Matthias Blüher, "Extended Longevity and Insulin Signaling in Adipose Tissue," *Experimental Gerontology* 40, no. 11 (2005).

4. Sarcopenia is an easily prevented condition of aging. Timothy J. Doherty, "Invited Review: Aging and Sarcopenia," *Journal of Applied Physiology* 95 (2003): 1717–27. But, it is more important to be strong than to have a lot of muscle mass; see Anne B. Newman et al., "Strength, But Not Muscle Mass, Is Associated with Mortality in the Health, Aging and Body Composition Study Cohort," *Journals of Gerontology, Series A* 61A, no. 1 (2006): 72–7.

5. Keep free radical damage at bay. See Wulf Dröge, "Oxidative Aging and Insulin Receptor Signaling," *Journals of Gerontology, Series A* 60A, no. 11 (2005): 1376–85; and Jeffrey G. Ault and David A. Lawrence, "Glutathione Distribution in Normal and Oxidatively Stressed Cells," *Experimental Cell Research* 285, no. 1 (2003): 9–14. Shigetada Furukawa et al., "Increased Oxidative Stress in Obesity and Its Impact on Metabolic Syndrome," *Journal of Clinical Investigation* 114, no. 12 (2004): 1752–61.
Oxidation (ROS damage) plays a large role in cell death because a large oxidative stress triggers the cell death program, as shown by Vladimir P. Skulachev and Valter D. Longo, "Aging as a Mitochondria-Mediated Atavistic Program: Can Aging Be Switched Off?" *Annals of the New York Academy of Sciences* 1057 (2005): 145–64. When they say it is an atavistic program, they mean that it is very old, a throwback to an earlier time, and may not be useful today. Our mitochondria are former bacteria that were incorporated into cells as protection against oxygen damage. They are the fuel cells that power us, but

they still have their atavistic attitude, forged eons ago. If we fail to protect them from oxidation, they may abandon ship (execute their death program) and leave us lacking in energy. Every cell in our body has its own DNA and its own interest to serve. The magic of life is only sustained when all these competing interests form a bond of cooperation.

6. Autophagy, the consumption of damaged proteins during a fast, is something I use as an antiaging strategy. I let it happen following my exercise by delaying my meal for about an hour afterward. See Wei-Lien Yen and Daniel J. Klionskty, "How to Live Long and Prosper: Autophagy, Mitochondria, and Aging," *Physiology* 23 (2008): 248–63. Exercise in a fasted state promotes autophagy and high protein turnover, which is a key factor in aging, as shown in Nektarious Tavernarakis and Monica Driscoll, "Caloric Restriction and Lifespan: A Role for Protein Turnover?" *Mechanisms of Ageing and Development* 125 (2002): 215–29.

Further Reading

My primary references are provided in the Notes section. If you are interested in further readings, I offer a list of some of my research that may deepen your understanding of the key ideas in the book. A complete bibliography is available on my Web site, www.arthurdevany.com.

The act of willpower costs energy and depletes glucose.

See Matthew T. Gailliot and Roy F. Baumeister, "The Physiology of Willpower: Linking Blood Glucose to Self-Control," *Personality and Social Psychology Review* 11 (2007): 303–27; and Huiyuan Zheng and Hans-Rudi Berthoud, "Neural Systems Controlling the Drive to Eat: Mind versus Metabolism," *Physiology* 23, no. 2 (2008): 75–83.

Fat secretes hormones and signaling molecules that affect insulin resistance, immunity, and inflammation.

See Barbara Antuna-Puente et al., "Adipokines: The Missing Link between Insulin Resistance and Obesity," *Diabetes and Metabolism* 34 (2008): 2–11; Pietro A Tataranni and Emilio Ortega, "A Burning Question: Does an Adipokine-Induced Activation of the Immune System Mediate the Effect of Overnutrition on Type 2 Diabetes?" *Diabetes* 54 (2005): 917–927; and Kathryn E. Wellen and Gökhan S. Hotamisligil, "Inflammation, Stress, and Diabetes," *Journal of Clinical Investigation* 115, no. 5 (2005): 1111–9. See also the positive effects of exercise on the hormones secreted by fat in Jason R. Berggen, Matthew W. Hulver, and Joseph A. Houmard, "Fat as an Endocrine Organ: Influence of Exercise," *Journal of Applied Physiology* 99 (2005): 757–64.

Does glucose restriction or calorie restriction increase longevity?

A good deal of aging research has focused on the insulin-IGF-1 pathway, implicating insulin as a key component of the aging pathways. Since insulin is deeply involved in glucose metabolism and storage, this suggests that glucose may be an important signal of the aging mechanisms. The insulin-IGF-1 pathway is ancient and exists in most organisms. When nutrients are abundant, the insulin-IGF signaling (IIS) pathway promotes growth and energy storage but shortens life span; see Meng C. Wang, Dirk Bohmann, and Heinrich Jasper, "JNK Extends Life Span and Limits Growth by Antagonizing Cellular and Organism-Wide Responses to Insulin Signaling," *Cell* 121 (2005): 115–25.

On how ancient this pathway is, see Michelangela Barbieri et al., "Insulin/IGF-I-Signaling Pathway: An Evolutionarily Conserved Mechanism of Longevity from Yeast to Humans," *American Journal of Physiology—Endocrinology and Metabolism* 285 (2003): E1064–71.

Dramatic new results that directly implicate glucose in longevity can be found in Seung-Jae Lee, Coleen T. Murphy, and Cynthia Kenyon, "Glucose Shortens the Life Span of *C. elegans* by Downregulating DAF-16/FOXO Activity and Aquaporin Gene Expression," *Cell Metabolism* 10 (2009): 379–91. This important article caused the researchers to drop sugars and simple starches from their diets immediately following their discovery, which is summarized in "Certain Proteins Extend Life Span in Worms by 30 Percent," ScienceDaily, www.sciencedaily.com/releases/2010/06/100616133319.htm.

Following the team's results for worms is another finding, by University of Alabama at Birmingham researchers, that in humans "restricting consumption of glucose, the most common dietary sugar, can extend the life of healthy human-lung cells and speed the death of precancerous human-lung cells, reducing cancer's spread and growth rate." See "Calorie Intake Linked to Cell Lifespan, Cancer Development," ScienceDaily, www.sciencedaily.com/releases/2009/12/091217183053.htm.

Further support for glucose restriction is in the remarkable finding that switching metabolism to glycolysis, of the sort stimulated by intense exercise, may induce the longevity effects of chronic caloric restriction in yeast and other organisms that share the same pathways activated by caloric restriction (humans share those pathways). See Min Wei et al., "Tor1/Sch9-Regulated Carbon Source Substitution Is as Effective as Calorie Restriction in Life Span Extension," *PLoS Genetics* 5, no. 5 (2009).

I find it very satisfying to have been applying both these ideas—glucose restriction and exhaustion of muscle glycogen—to my own life for over 2 decades, long before they were discovered in the lab.

The persisting alteration of gene expression following those holiday "I'll just do it this one time" binging episodes is described in Assam El-Osta et al., "Transient High Glucose Causes Persistent Epigenetic Changes and Altered Gene Expression during Subsequent Normoglycemia," *Journal of Experimental Medicine* 205, no. 10 (2008): 2409–17. This is the mechanism behind the metabolic memory that I had found in my first wife's blood sugars following a big bowl of spaghetti or an episode of low blood glucose.

Stress resistance through calorie restriction is discussed in Byung P. Yu and Hae Young Chung, "Stress Resistance by Caloric Restriction for Longevity," *Annals of the New York Academy of Sciences* 928 (2001): 39–47.

Oxidation, obesity, and aging.

See Jeffrey G. Ault and David A. Lawrence, "Glutathione Distribution in Normal and Oxidatively Stressed Cells," *Experimental Cell Research* 285, no. 1 (2003): 9–14; and Shigetada Furukawa et al., "Increased Oxidative Stress in Obesity and Its Impact on Metabolic Syndrome," *Journal of Clinical Investigation* 114, no. 12 (2004): 1752–61.

The relationship of inflammation to loss of muscle mass in aging is reviewed in A. M. Solomon and P. M. G. Bouloux, "Modifying Muscle Mass—the Endocrine Perspective," *Journal of Endocrinology* 191 (2006): 349–60. Their abstract is almost pure drama: Aging is associated with inflammatory chronic conditions such as obesity, cardiovascular disease, insulin resistance, and arthritis. Sarcopenia—muscle loss with aging—is multifactorial, with contributing factors that may include loss of motor neuron input, changes in anabolic hormones, decreased intake of dietary protein, and decline in physical activity. Research findings suggest that sarcopenia is a smoldering inflammatory state driven by cytokines and oxidative stress.

Oxidation (ROS damage) plays a large role in cell death because a large oxidative stress triggers the cell death program, as shown by Vladimir P. Skulachev and Valter D. Longo, "Aging as a Mitochondria-Mediated Atavistic Program: Can Aging Be Switched Off?" *Annals of the New York Academy of Sciences* 1057 (2005): 145–64.

Reinterpreting energy balance and thermodynamics.

Weight gain is driven by elevated insulin; increased appetite and reduced movement are the results of weight gain, not its cause. See Robert Lustig, "Childhood Obesity: Behavioral Aberration or Biochemical Drive? Reinterpreting the First Law of Thermodynamics," *Nature Clinical Practice Endocrinology and Metabolism* 2, no. 8 (2006): 447–58.

Weight loss shows similar effects that, on first glance, defy the first law of thermodynamics (weight gain or loss equals energy in minus energy out). But a deeper look at energy expenditure induced by protein versus carbohydrate shows that higher-protein diets have a metabolic advantage; so one loses more weight on the higher-protein diet. See Richard D. Feinman and Eugene J. Fine, "Nonequilibrium Thermodynamics and Energy Efficiency in Weight Loss Diets," *Theoretical Biology and Medical Modelling* 4 (2007), www.tbiomed.com/content/4/1/27.

I show that energy balance is stochastic and that an evolutionary stable energy strategy for our ancestors required that they eat, on average, more than they expend in energy; see Arthur De Vany, "Why We Get Fat" (1998), available at www.arthurdevany.com. I call this the "lazy overeater" strategy in the text.

Not all calories are equal. Questioning that a calorie is really a calorie is becoming serious research, as in Anssi H. Manninen, "Is a Calorie Really a Calorie? Metabolic Advantage of Low-Carbohydrate Diets," *Journal of the International Society of Sports Nutrition* 83, no. 6 (2004): 1442–3.

The crowning piece in the ongoing work to recast homeostasis and equilibrium thermodynamics—which, in my view, have impeded real understanding of diet and exercise—is the careful modeling of energy flux in the human organism as a far-from-equilibrium process in Feinman and Fine, "Nonequilibrium Thermodynamics and Energy Efficiency," which contains an extensive review of the experimental evidence, and sets the results into the nonequilibrium model to more or less completely refute the old view that "a calorie is a calorie."

It is carbohydrate that provides the signal metabolism relies on to store or burn fat, which is convincingly shown in the clever experiment done by S. Klein and R. R. Wolfe, who show that "carbohydrate restriction, not the presence of a negative energy balance, is responsible for initiating the metabolic response to fasting." See Klein and Wolfe, "Carbohydrate Restriction Regulates the Adaptive Response to Fasting," *American Journal of Physiology* 262, no. 5, pt. 1 (1992): E631–6.

Exercise.

Short-duration, high-intensity exercise improves insulin sensitivity, gene expression, and muscle. See John A. Barbraj et al., "Extremely Short Duration High Intensity Interval Training Substantially Improves Insulin Action in Young Healthy Males," *BioMedCentral Endocrine Disorders* 9, no. 3 (2009): 1–21; and Maria A. Fiatarone Singh et al., "Insulin-Like Growth Factor I in Skeletal Muscle After Weight-Lifting Exercise in Frail Elders," *American Journal of Physiology—Endocrinology and Metabolism* 277 (1999): E135–43.

Exercising with low carbohydrate stores in the muscles, something that is almost anathema to runners and body builders, improves the genetic response to exercise. Low carbohydrate stores in muscle improve gene expression response to exercise. Katrien De Bock et al., "Effect of Training in the Fasted State on Metabolic Responses during Exercise with Carbohydrate Intake," *Journal of Applied Physiology* 104 (2008): 1045–55. Exercise releases lactate and growth hormone.

The metabolic effects of high- or low-intensity exercise are examined in N. E. Felsing, "Effect of Low and High Intensity Exercise on Circulating Growth Hormone in Men," *Journal of Clinical Endocrinology and Metabolism* 75 (1992): 157–62. High-intensity exercise produces a better growth hormone response.

The safety of high-intensity exercise is examined in Darren E. R. Warburton et al., "Effectiveness of High-Intensity Interval Training for the Rehabilitation of Patients with Coronary Artery Disease," *American Journal of Cardiology* 95, no. 9 (2005): 1–5.

The importance of growth hormone to the heart and other systems is illustrated in A. S. Khan et al., "Growth Hormone, Insulin-Like Growth Factor-1 and the Aging Cardiovascular System," *Cardiovascular Research* 54, no. 1 (2002): 25–35. High-intensity weight lifting is the premier releaser of growth hormone.

An excellent book on high-intensity, intermittent exercise is Doug McDuff and John Little's *Body by Science* (New York: McGraw-Hill, 2009).

Adequate protein intake is essential.

See Anna E. Thalaker-Mercer et al., "Inadequate Protein Intake Affects Skeletal Muscle Transcript Profiles in Older Humans," *Physiological Genomics* 85, no. 5 (2007): 1344–52. See also M. M. Porter, A. A. Vandervoort, and J. Lexell, "Aging of Human Muscle: Structure, Function and Adaptability,"

Scandinavian Journal of Medicine and Science in Sports 5, no. 3 (1995): 129–42; and H. Pilegaard et al., "Substrate Availability and Transcriptional Regulation of Metabolic Genes in Human Skeletal Muscle during Recovery from Exercise," *Metabolism* 54 (2005): 1048–55. And see Micah J. Drummond et al., "Expression of Growth-Related Genes in Young and Old Human Skeletal Muscle Following an Acute Stimulation of Protein Synthesis," *Journal of Applied Physiology* 106 (2009): 1403–11.

Having a complete intake of amino acids is important for controlling the appetite because the brain senses the lack of any essential amino acid and promotes more food intake to secure the missing or deficient amino acid. Methionine is one of the most important amino acids, as it is essential to the formation of all proteins. Methionine occurs in naturally high levels in foods such as sesame seeds, Brazil nuts, wheat germ, fish, and meats. The New Evolution Diet is relatively low in calories and assures a balanced amino acid profile. According to research, this combination may reduce aging; see "Balancing Protein Intake, Not Cutting Calories, May Be Key to Long Life," ScienceDaily, December 6, 2009, www.sciencedaily.com/releases/2009/12/091202131622.htm.

Obesity, metabolic syndrome, and testosterone.

See Michael Zitzmann, "Testosterone Deficiency, Insulin Resistance and the Metabolic Syndrome," *Nature Reviews Endocrinology* 5 (2009): 673–81. On the effect of visceral fat on metabolism, see Ellen W. Demerath et al., "Visceral Adiposity and Its Anatomical Distribution as Predictors of the Metabolic Syndrome and Cardiometabolic Risk Factor Levels," *American Journal of Clinical Nutrition* 88, no. 5 (2008): 1263–71.

Body composition and aging.

Research tells us that loss of muscle mass is associated with aging and may even be what aging really is. One review summarizes the connection thusly: "Sarcopenia is associated with a reduction in muscle mass and strength occurring with normal aging, associated with a reduction in motor unit number and atrophy of muscle fibers, especially the type IIb fibers [the fastest fibers]. The loss of muscle mass with aging is clinically important because it leads to diminished strength and exercise capacity." See David R. Thomas, "Loss of Skeletal Muscle Mass in Aging: Examining the Relationship of Starvation, Sarcopenia and Cachexia," *Clinical Nutrition* 26, no. 4 (2007): 389–99.

Exercise in a fasted state promotes autophagy and high protein turnover, which is a key factor in aging, as shown by Nektarious Tavernarakis and Monica Driscoll, "Caloric Restriction and Lifespan: A Role for Protein Turnover?" *Mechanisms of Ageing and Development* 125 (2002): 215–29.

It may be that the many benefits of calorie or glucose restriction involve the effect of body composition on aging. Researchers from the University of Alabama at Birmingham have shown that a lean body composition is protective against cancer and metabolic syndrome. See "Body Composition May Be Key Player in Controlling Cancer Risks," ScienceDaily, January 3, 2007, www.sciencedaily.com/releases/2007/01/070102104108.htm.

Obesity, metabolic syndrome, and brain function and health.

See Fernando Gómez-Pinilla, "Brain Foods: The Effects of Nutrients on Brain Function," *Nature Reviews Neuroscience* 9 (2008): 568–78; and Werner Kern, Jan Born, and Horst L. Fehm, "Role of Insulin in Alzheimer's Disease: Approaches Emerging from Basic Animal Research and Neurocognitive Studies in Humans," *Drug Development Research* 56, no. 3 (2002): 511–25. Does carbohydrate help or impede brain function? See E. L. Gibson, "Carbohydrates and Mental Function: Feeding or Impeding the Brain?" *Nutrition Bulletin* 32, no. S1 (2007): 71–83.

If you read only one article about bad food and brain function, make it Robert H. Lustig's "How Our Western Environment Starves Kids' Brains," *Pediatric Annals* 35, no. 12 (2006): 905–7.

Stress.

A wonderfully written, science-drenched but readable discussion of stress is Robert Sapolski's *Why Zebras Don't Get Ulcers,* 3rd ed. (New York: Henry Holt and Company, 2004). How stress, inflammation, and metabolism are intertwined is covered in Kathryn E. Wellen and Gökhan S. Hotamisligil, "Inflammation, Stress, and Diabetes," *Journal of Clinical Investigation* 115, no. 5 (2005): 1111–9; and Mary F. Dallman et al., "Minireview: Glucocorticoids—Food Intake, Abdominal Obesity, and Wealthy Nations in 2004," *Endocrinology* 145, no. 6 (2004): 2633–8.

The failure of feedback loops to control stress is shown in Mary F. Dallman et al., "Stress, Feedback and Facilitation in the Hypothalamo-Pituitary-Adrenal Axis," *Journal of Neuroendocrinology* 4, no. 5 (1992): 517–26.

Exercise is good for the brain.

See Carl W. Cotman and Nicole C. Berchtold, "Exercise: A Behavioral Intervention to Enhance Brain Health and Plasticity," *Trends in Neurosciences* 25
(2002): 295–301. I do have a problem with them calling exercise an
"intervention," but I always feel better after exercising, and it is because
of the way exercise or play releases brain neurotrophic factor (a kind of
growth hormone for neurons).

Aging.

"Can You Really Extend Your Life?" Chapter 8 of *Closer to Truth: Challenging
Conventional Wisdom*, edited by Robert Lawrence Kuhn (New York:
McGraw-Hill, 2000): 111–121, contains the transcript of the segment of
the show I appeared in where I questioned the progress in extending life
in the face of the declining health and increasing obesity of the world's
population.

Is aging really an evolved mechanism rather than just the accumulation of
damage? I think the answer is yes. Starting with the mitochondria—
those energy furnaces in our cells—one of my favorite scientists, Vladimir Skulachev, takes this topic to new heights. See Vladimir P. Skulachev
and Valter D. Longo, "Aging as a Mitochondria-Mediated Atavistic Program: Can Aging Be Switched Off?" *Annals of the New York Academy of
Sciences* 1057 (2005): 145–64.

Skulachev shows why he is one of my favorite researchers again in this tour
de force article on a genetically programmed death program: Skulachev,
"The Programmed Death Phenomena, Aging, and the Samurai Law of
Biology," *Experimental Gerontology* 36, no. 7 (2001): 995–1024. My
approach to health and aging affects every one of the key death programs noted in the article in a way that seems to be favorable.

Strengthening the point that aging *is* a loss of body composition, which I
make in regard to inflammation, is R. N. Baumgartner, "Body Composition in Healthy Aging," *Annals of the New York Academy of Sciences* 904
(2000): 437–48.

Reactive oxygen species damage muscle and contribute to the loss of muscle
with aging, particularly those fast-twitch fibers; see Stefania Fulle et al.,
"The Contribution of Reactive Oxygen Species to Sarcopenia and Muscle
Ageing," *Experimental Gerontology* 39 (2004): 17–24.

To be lean and have high insulin sensitivity are keys to living long and well,
as shown in Nora Klöting and Matthias Blüher, "Extended Longevity

and Insulin Signaling in Adipose Tissue, *Experimental Gerontology* 40, no. 11 (2005).

Exercise is the fountain of youth. It reverses the expression of genes associated with aging; see Simon Melov et al., "Resistance Exercise Reverses Aging in Human Skeletal Muscle," *PLoS ONE* 2, no. 5 (2007). The authors note that "following a period of resistance exercise training in older adults, we found that age-associated transcriptome expression changes were reversed, implying a restoration of a youthful expression profile."

Diet.

The power of nutrition to shape evolution and the importance of fatty acids in human evolution are beautifully exposited in Michael Crawford and David Marsh, *Nutrition and Evolution* (New Canaan, Connecticut: Keats Publishing, 1995).

Consumption of marine-based foods in human evolution is discussed in Nuno Bicho and Jonathan Haws, "At the Land's End: Marine Resources and the Importance of Fluctuations in the Coastline in the Prehistoric Hunter-Gatherer Economy of Portugal," *Quaternary Science Review* 27, no. 23–24 (2008): 2166–75.

The effects of consuming a hunter-gather diet are superior to the benefits of the Mediterranean diet, as shown in Lynda A. Frassetto et al., "Metabolic and Physiologic Improvements from Consuming a Paleolithic, Hunter-Gatherer Type Diet," *European Journal of Clinical Nutrition* 63 (2009): 947–55.

A very-low-carbohydrate diet profoundly alters the fatty acid profile favorably and reduces inflammation. See C. E. Forsyth et al., "Comparison of Low Fat and Low Carbohydrate Diets on Circulating Fatty Acid Composition and Markers of Inflammation," *Lipids* 43, no. 1 (2008): 65–77.

A telling reassessment of the low-fat diet as a treatment for diabetes and obesity is found in Anthony Accurso et al., "Dietary Carbohydrate Restriction in Type 2 Diabetes Mellitus and Metabolic Syndrome: Time for a Critical Appraisal," *Nutrition and Metabolism* 5, no. 9 (2008): 1438–52. In the article, experiments are summarized showing that carbohydrate-restricted diets are at least as effective for weight loss as low-fat diets and that the substitution of fat for carbohydrate is generally beneficial for risk of cardiovascular disease. These beneficial effects of carbohydrate restriction do not require weight loss. Finally, the point is reiterated that carbohydrate restriction improves all the features of metabolic syndrome.

Carbohydrate restriction shifts fuel sources from glucose and fatty acids to fatty acids and ketones, and carbohydrate-restricted diets lead to appetite reduction, weight loss, and improvement in markers of cardiovascular disease, as shown in Eric C. Westman et al., "Low-Carbohydrate Nutrition and Metabolism," *American Journal of Clinical Nutrition* 86, no. 2 (2007): 276–84; and Eric C. Westman and Mary C. Vernon, "Has Carbohydrate-Restriction Been Forgotten as a Treatment for Diabetes Mellitus? A Perspective on the ACCORD Study Design," *Nutrition and Metabolism* 5, no. 10 (2008): 1–2. See also Douglas Paddon-Jones et al., "Protein, Weight Management, and Satiety," *American Journal of Clinical Nutrition* 87, no. 5 (2008): S1558–61.

Low-carbohydrate diets are comparable or better than traditional low-fat, high-carbohydrate diets for weight reduction, improvement in the poor fatty acid control of diabetes, and metabolic syndrome, as well as the control of blood pressure, postmeal blood-glucose control, and insulin level. This is shown in Surender K. Arora and Samy I. McFarlane, "The Case for Low Carbohydrate Diets in Diabetes Management," *Nutrition and Metabolism* 2, no. 16 (2005).

An unusually long follow-up period for a diet study of 44 months on a low-carbohydrate diet showed steady improvement in body weight and glucose control, as reported in Jørgen Vesti Nielsen and Eva Joensson, "Low-Carbohydrate Diet in Type 2 Diabetes: Stable Improvement of Bodyweight and Glycemic Control during 44 Months Follow-Up," *Nutrition and Metabolism* 4, no. 14 (2008).

See also a stronger point defining metabolic syndrome as the *response* to carbohydrate in Jeff S. Volek and Richard D. Feinman, "Carbohydrate Restriction Improves the Features of Metabolic Syndrome. Metabolic Syndrome May Be Defined by the Response to Carbohydrate Restriction," *Nutrition and Metabolism* 2, no. 31 (2005): 1–17.

The role of insulin in food preference and weight is clarified in P. A. Velasquez-Mieyer et al., "Suppression of Insulin Secretion Is Associated with Weight Loss and Altered Macronutrient Intake and Preference in a Subset of Obese Adults," *International Journal of Obesity and Related Metabolic Disorders* 27, no. 3 (2003): 219–26.

Loren Cordain's *The Paleo Diet: Lose Weight and Get Healthy by Eating the Food You Were Designed to Eat* (New York: John Wiley and Sons, 2002) thoroughly explains the eating patterns of hunter-gatherers and shows how to adapt their foods to a modern diet.

Gary Taubes's *Good Calories, Bad Calories* (New York: Alfred A. Knopf, 2008) is an excellent review of the diet literature and a challenge to the accepted view on weight control and disease.

Competition within.

One of the most original and important theories of internal competition is
Achim Peters et al., "The Selfish Brain: Competition for Energy
Resources," *Neuroscience and Biobehavioral Reviews* 28, no. 2 (2004):
143–80. This is almost straight economics, with the hormonal and neural actors all put into play to see.

Peters and his coauthors ingeniously apply selfish-brain theory to the problem
of obesity in Peters et al., "Causes of Obesity: Looking Beyond the Hypothalamus," *Progress in Neurobiology* 81 (2007): 61–88. I had stumbled
upon the economic model—naturally, since I am an economist—as we
worked through my wife's diabetes. I had only a few hints of all the
complex metabolic pathways involved at the time, yet we had worked
out the same strategy.

The energy-on-demand concept that I utilized to shift our diet toward low-
carbohydrate, low-glycemic foods and to rely more on internal sources of
glucose for the brain is elegantly demonstrated in this important article:
Pellerin and Magistretti, "Food for Thought; Challenging the Dogmas,"
Journal of Cerebral Blood Flow and Metabolism; vol 23 (2003): 1282–6.

Together the Peters and Magistretti articles, and the many that cite and expand
their models, support the economic model of internal competition and
cooperation in human metabolism and health. It is not so strange that an
economist figured this out, as it turns out to be an economic problem.

Fuels compete for utilization inside the body, and insulin resistance is a strategy the brain uses to protect its supply of glucose. A discussion of this
competition and the importance of insulin resistance is in Ping Wang
and Edwin C. M. Mariman, "Insulin Resistance in an Energy-Centered
Perspective," *Physiology and Behavior* 94 (2008): 198–205.

Refer to Vladimir Skulachev's "The Programmed Death Phenomena" and Skulachev and Longo's "Aging as a Mitochondria-Mediated Atavistic Program," noted under "Aging," to see how cell death programs help in
managing the competition within. The abstract from his Samurai law
of biology reveals the need for a death program for damaged or rogue
cells: "Analysis of the programmed death phenomena from mitochondria (mitoptosis) to whole organisms (phenoptosis) clearly shows that
suicide programs are inherent at various levels of organization of living
systems. Such programs perform very important functions, purifying
(i) cells from damaged (or unwanted for other reasons) organelles, (ii)
tissues from unwanted cells, (iii) organisms from organs transiently

appearing during ontogenesis, and (iv) communities of organisms from unwanted individuals."

Brain and body compete for fuel and nutrients and, in the obese, the brain loses some of its essential supplies, and parts of it shrink; see Cyrus A. Raji et al., "Brain Structure and Obesity," *Human Brain Mapping* 31, no. 3 (2009): 353–64.

Complexity, fractals, and chaos.

An early article linking complexity of the heartbeat to aging, which uses chaos theory and fractals to measure complexity, is Sirkku M. Pikkujämsä et al., "Cardiac Interbeat Interval Dynamics from Childhood to Senescence Comparison of Conventional and New Measures Based on Fractals and Chaos Theory," *Circulation* 100 (1999): 393–9.

New models of human physiology and metabolism are expanding the idea of homeostasis to the wider, dynamical systems point of view. Recognition of the dynamic nature of regulatory processes challenges the prevailing view of homeostasis, which asserts that all healthy cells, tissues, and organs maintain static or steady-state conditions in their internal environment. The new view, and the view I take in this book, is to rely on interacting, complex, dynamical notions of sustaining life far from equilibrium. Lewis A. Lipsitz points to this new way of looking at living systems in his "Dynamics of Stability: The Physiologic Basis of Functional Health and Frailty," *Journal of Gerontology, Series A* 57A, no. 3 (2002): B115–25.

A survey of the applications of fractal dynamics to disease and physiology is Ary L. Goldberger et al., "Fractal Dynamics in Physiology: Alterations with Disease and Aging," *Proceedings of the National Academy of Sciences* 99, suppl. no. 1 (2002): 2466–72. They say that the nonlinear regulatory systems are operating far from equilibrium and that maintaining constancy is not the goal of physiologic control.

Bruce West's *Where Medicine Went Wrong: Rediscovering the Path to Complexity* (Singapore: World Scientific, 2006) shows the errors that result from considering the body to be a simple system, even multiple simple systems, and offers a way of replacing traditional physiology with a fractal physiology based on complexity.

Dietary supplements.

On the use of melatonin, see Mónica Kotler et al., "Melatonin Increases Gene Expression for Antioxidant Enzymes in Rat Brain Cortex," *Journal of Pineal Research* 24, no. 2 (1998): 83–9.

Index